The Other Side

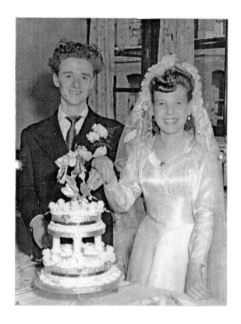

A True Story of Love Pain, Sacrifice and Hope

John Carrigan

Published by
Chipmunkapublishing
PO Box 6872
Brentwood
Essex CM13 1ZT
United Kingdom

http://www.chipmunkapublishing.com

The Other Side Of Harry

This book is about the dark illness of Schizophrenia which continues to tear people apart even today, and about the legacy of demons it leaves behind for the family's to deal with, demons which take years to conquer…if they ever truly can be conquered.
But this book is also about love, sacrifice and hope, which against all the odds were the only things which brought my family through hell, to the brightness of today, and the hope of tomorrow.

THE PHOENIX MUST BURN BEFORE IT CAN RISE, RENEWED BY THE FLAME WHICH SAUGHT TO DESTROY IT

Dedicated to Margaret Carrigan (my mum) the unsung hero, who got me through to today and gave so much.

TOP OF THE WORLD MA.

John Carrigan

The Beginning

Our story begins with the birth of Henry Daniel Carrigan on 20 April 1926, at No 17 Jane Street in Southwark, London, born to parents John Carrigan and Amelia Ward who at that time were not married. My father Henry (who we will call Harry for the rest of this book) was one of eight children, four boys and four girls, the youngest of which Eileen died when she was only seven years of age.

The other important birth in that same year was that of Margaret Lillian Healy, born on 18 January 1926 at No 6 Gabriel Street in Southwark, London, born to parents John Healey and Margaret Healey. My mother Margaret (who everyone called Maggie) was one of ten children, three boys and seven girls.

My dads family moved into Gabriel St where my mums family already lived, which meant that all the children ended up going to the same school together, it was at that school where my parents first met. All the Healey children got to know all the Carrigan children (which sounds like the beginning of a Fairy story), but in the pre war days the close knit street communities really did get on a lot like the Walton's, and people really did not bother to lock their doors. The World was a different place then.

In his youth my dad was quite the ladies man, with many girls trying to win his attention, which he gloried in to the point of arrogance, my mum on the other hand, although a very beautiful girl, talented acrobat and tap dancer, was quiet and turned down the many boys who also flocked around her, because as she told me many times, she only really ever had eyes for Harry.

In those early times just before the war many working class children left school very young, at around fourteen years of age, and so it was with Harry and Maggie. They managed to get a job together sorting through mountains of old rags and clothes, my dads job was to stuff them into big bins and then jump them down, my parents were also very active in their respective hobbies, dad took up boxing and football, he also started to dabble with the piano, not in any classical sense but in the grand old tradition of the pub sing along, he later grew into a very talented pianist. My mum's hobby of acrobatics and dancing led her to join a respected dance troop called Madam Terrie's, she loved to tap dance and really wanted it to be her career, which lead her to audition for a very well known dance troop who had been on the bill at the London Palladium. Young Margaret was over the Moon when she won her place, she was going to be one of the twenty tiny tappers dance troop which would have taken her into a life of show business. But it was not meant to be, the war broke out and all normal life came to an end and nobody knew for how long. Dancing became a thing of the past as surviving became top on everyone's list.

Harry was called up and my mum's dancers were disbanded while everyone fought just to survive. I was told many War stories by my parents, of life sleeping in the underground stations, of German planes machine gunning the hop picking huts in Kent because they thought they were Army barracks, and of watching the battle of Britain live over head as my parents families picked fruit and hops on their annual holiday during 1940, the only holiday many Londoners ever had, including myself up until my early teens. But for my dad the war held a bitter memory, one I did not find out about for many years. My dad was enlisted into the Royal Fusiliers, and from what I could gather did his training well, but when it came time for him to go over sea's to fight, he along with his best army buddy deserted, I never got to know the reason why, but from the man I came to know in later life I do not think it was because of fear alone, but I would not have blamed him if it was. Like so many others he was thrown into that terrible war while still only a boy himself. After deserting his own mother would have nothing to do with him so my mum's mother (a lovely woman by all accounts) hid him and looked after him until she persuaded Harry to give himself up. When he did this he was promptly court marshalled and sent to a harsh military prison, if he had deserted after he had gone abroad he could well have been shot. My mum and her family stuck by him and were his only light at that dark time, maybe a forewarning of things to come.

Eventually the war ended and Harry served his time, I am not sure just how long, but it was not more than a couple of years or so, (which must have seemed a lifetime to him) and when he returned to the World outside, his loyal girl Maggie was waiting for him. They finally went steady (as they said in those innocent days) and were married not long after. Their early married life was a happy time for them in post war England, full of the promise of tomorrow.

Harry boy (as a lot of people called him) worked as a lorry driver by day and was the star attraction on the piano in the Fountain pub at The Elephant and Castle by night. My mum and dad moved into No. 27 Oswin Street, which was still in view of Gabriel St where they had grown up, to begin their new life together and think about planning a family. No 27 was a typical London house in a typical London street, it had four floors, one toilet, and no hot water, which became the only home I knew until my late teens (still with that one toilet and no hot water). My parents had the top two rooms and various members of my dad's family had the rest of the house. My dad's mother lived on the ground floor and also acted as the land lady collecting the rent from the rest of the tenants, this left one of my dad's sisters (Mary) to occupy the middle floors, not quite the Walton's but close.

A Child Is Born

On September 27th 1950 my sister Susan (Sue) was born, and I am sure that mum and dad were over the Moon.

After asking my sister about the days before my time, She told me that her first memory was of a coal fire in the bedroom, watching the flames flickering while going to sleep, her dad, Harry coming home from playing the piano with lots of coins which people had dropped into his collection hat, and jellied eels with vinegar and pepper, which Sue loved from an early age. They were happy times for my family, there was not a lot of money around but with my dad's job on the railway and his coins from playing his piano it was enough, my sister said she wanted for nothing. But after her sixth birthday her world would change for ever. On the 4th of April 1957 I was born, Paul Henry John Carrigan, a healthy nine pound bouncing baby boy. For reasons I will go into later in this book, for most of my life I have been called John, but on all official documents I am still Paul, which can get confusing at times.

When Darkness Comes

The dark times really began about seven weeks after I was born, when the other side of Harry first showed itself.

We were about to go hopping (hop picking) in Kent, as our families had always done and I was lying on the sofa in my carry cot with not a care in the world as babies are inclined to do, and my mum was sitting on one side of an open fireplace with my dad sitting on the other side. My mum told me that my father had been a bit off that day, quiet, with a strange smile which crossed his face from time to time, but apart from that it was a normal day. While they were sitting by the fire Harry suddenly leaned forward to her and said, "you would never leave me would you my angel", my mum was shocked and said "what"! He again quietly said, "You are my angel and you would never leave me would you". My mum told me this was out of the blue, so she said "don't be stupid of course I wouldn't". Harry stood up and went over to her, kissed her on top of the head and stroked her face saying, "you're my angel and we are always going to be together". What my mother didn't know was that as one of my father's hands stroked her face, the other one was reaching for the poker which was part of a set by the fire place.

Without warning the man she loved lifted up the poker and smashed it down onto my mothers head, this began a desperate fight for life, as

The Other Side Of Harry

Harry rained blow after blow down on her. After the first terrible blow my mum had managed to get to her feet, she told me she remembered the white light as the poker struck her, she remembered the thick jam like blood running into her eyes, and she remembered fighting, fighting for her life. Punching, kicking, clawing, screaming all the way around the sofa trying to get to the door as blow after blow continued to fall onto her shattered head, and all the while I lay oblivious to all of this, only feet away on the sofa. The door to our front room had a brass door knob which always took a few turns to open due to the fact that it was loose, but my mum said that just for that one time when she finally reached it, the door opened on her first desperate try. She carried on fighting her now crazed Harry down the stairs, still screaming all the while. The rest of the house had gathered further down on the lower floors listening, but were too afraid to go up those stairs. We do not know how she did it but my mum fought for her life down many flights of stairs and into the hallway screaming "my baby my baby", as family members stood frozen in disbelief at the horrific sight of my blood-soaked mother staggering past them.

I obviously have no memories of this terrible day but my sister does, so I will let her tell it in her own words. (Sue) I had a little kitten which my mum had bought for me and I was waiting down stairs by the street door for my mum, dad and newly arrived baby brother John, I remember being excited at going away and being allowed to bring my kitten with me. Suddenly I heard my auntie who lived on the second floor start to scream, as I looked into the hallway I saw my mother hanging on to the banisters, partly walking, partly falling down the stairs with blood pouring down her face. My auntie Mary was hanging on to her and calling for help, I can't explain to this day how I felt, but I started calling, "mummy mummy". The neighbour from next door brushed by and picked my mother up in his arms and rushed outside again, they then wrapped her head in towels and strapped her to a plank of wood on the sidecar of a motorbike before rushing her to the nearest hospital. My auntie was still screaming and ran into the downstairs kitchen. Even more horrific to me was the sight of my father who was calling, "Maggie Maggie", as he walked down the stairs with his arms stretched out in front of him, and blood spurting up the walls from gaping wounds in his wrists which he had slashed 36 times, he thought he had killed the woman he loved, so he wanted to die too.

For my sister to see all of this at her young age must have left feelings inside her which I can only guess at, what a memory for a young girl to carry with her. My mum had multiple fractures to her skull which had been caused by at least eighteen blows from a poker, wielded by my now insane father, how did she survive…it could so easily have been me too.

With our mother in critical condition and my father sectioned into a secure ward beside her, it was left to my parents large families to look after my sister and I, but with my being a seven week old baby, it was not an easy task, and as soon as she was able my mum made sure she was back with us far sooner than she should have done for her own health (although she was still in Hospital for three months) but that was mum all over, never ever thinking of herself. Obviously the Police were involved because it was attempted murder, they wanted my mother to press charges and commit Harry to a mental institution for the rest of his life (or at least most of it) she was also told to go for a quick divorce right away. Now in my mums later years she cried and told my sister and I that she had been racked with guilt from that day forward for the two of us, because of the decision she made during that time. In her heart she still loved the man she married and could not bring herself to press charges and have him committed for life-or divorce him, which paved the way for all that was to come, in all our lives.

As I have said I have no memory of these earliest black years, so my sister will again fill in the blanks about what came next in the nightmare which was now our life.

(Sue) When mum came home I remember her crying and cuddling my brother and me saying, we will be ok, I know God's good. In the weeks to follow the woman we called Auntie Amy (from next door, who was no real relation) played a big part in our lives, she was always there for us and used to bring us food and help mum with money, as we were penniless. Mum couldn't get any money from the state and decided that she had to go to work; early morning cleaning was all she could fit in with looking after John and myself. I used to be taken to school, while Auntie Amy looked after John, later mum would pick me up from school with John in her arms and when we got home we used to have whatever mum could afford that day, it was never much, soup and potatoes and maybe biscuits. Aunt Mary and Uncle Elf (dad's sister and mum's brother) decided to move from 27 Oswin Street, they were frightened by the thought of Harry at some stage coming home (so much for family support). Dad also had a sister (Kitty) who owned a shop full of food and we used to get minimal stuff from her, on tick as they called it, which mum used to pay for when she herself got paid. But we stopped going to Aunt Kit because someone told mum that Kit's husband (Lenny) had said that we only went there to see what we could get for free, which was so untrue. Mum's sister Aunty Vi also had two shops (also full of food) and when we used to visit her mum might be given some tea, soup and maybe we would get some cake, which was a real treat, but mum did all of Aunt Vi's housework and got paid £1.00 per week.

We loved Aunt Vi but looking back on it, in mum's situation the whole family could have done so much more without making mum feel like the poor relation, which through no fault of her own she now was. But during those times another one of mum's sisters was of great help. Auntie Eady, she made sure that every now and again she would do her best to give us a helping hand, and every Christmas she would make sure the two of us at least had new clothes, but mum was the kind of person who found it almost impossible to accept any kind of charity. My sister told me that while dad was in hospital mum would take us to the pie and mash shop because she knew that we could buy a large bowl of mash with green gravy called liquor, which would be enough to fill us up. One day the owner noticed that this woman who always came in alone with her two children only ever ordered a bowl of mash and liquor, so without asking anything she brought over a load of pies and mash for us, and said don't worry this is on me, I know you don't have much money. Well my mum could not bring herself to ever go back into the pie shop in case the owner thought she only came in for some more free food. Mum's attitude of never asking anyone for help would last her whole life, and would not always be for the best, but sometimes when you have nothing, pride is all you can really call your own.

(Sue continues) The next step was going to see my father in Cain Hill hospital with mum and John.

We used to travel by train to Caulsdon South, get off at the station and walk to the hospital which seemed a long way to me, then a bus used to pick us up at the bottom of the hill (the hospital was like Dracula's castle at the top of a winding narrow road) I didn't like it much as there were some really strange people around. The hospital was massive, in acres of land, and when we got in It was sort of like a prison. Dad was in a locked ward and there were a great deal of male nurses sort of on guard, he looked dreadful but he still cuddled us all, they had given him shock treatment so he moved and talked very slowly. When it came time for us to leave, he cried and said he wanted to come home with us, I remember mum being very upset going home and leaving him.

As time went on things seemed to be ok but we didn't see much of dad because mum couldn't afford the train fare very often. I then started to become very stressed and had times when I couldn't breathe, If I saw the TV and somebody was dying, I used to think that I was dying too and start to panic. The doctor said it was how the whole thing had effected me, and it had to come out in some way, it was a kind of post traumatic stress and this went on for many months, but I did eventually get over it.

John was about 7 months old by now and they decided to let dad home for a weekend, we were all happy as doctors had seen him and told us he was on the mend. Little did we know, once my father got back home he wouldn't go back and made us virtual prisoners, we spent the whole weekend not allowed out. I was worried about mum because she didn't seem to be herself, but he had probably been saying things to her that I wasn't aware of, anyhow the next thing I remember was Auntie Amy from next door coming in and saying, "Hello Harry boy, getting ready to go back?" He told her in no uncertain terms to go and FUCK OFF, She left and phoned the hospital and our doctor (Radcliff) came out and chatted with him. As our doctor left he winked at my mum and very soon two male nurses and a policemen arrived to take my father back to hospital. Eventually it took five men and a straight jacket to control my dad, fortunately we all escaped to Nan's downstairs before he knew the rescue party was in the house. Poor mum was petrified, I was frightened but not that much, I suppose I didn't really grasp what was fully going on. Dad went away again and we continued to visit him, he was always very strange and hostile toward mum saying she was a spy for the government and didn't trust her. On one visit he seemed to be ok and asked me what I had done at the Brownies (like cub scouts, but for girls) I said I learnt to tie knots, then I sneezed and dad suddenly said, No Susan you mustn't listen to those people who tell you to send secret messages, he had obviously heard one in my innocent little sneeze.

Mum struggled on with no help from any of the family, they ceased to come near. Several times over the next two years dad escaped or was discharged from hospital and came home, we used to be really frightened because you never knew what to expect, sometimes he went back voluntarily, but more often than not Police were involved. One memory of the early days of dad's illness makes me shudder when I think of it now. He went through a phase of taking me on long walks at night over the bridges of London. We would get to a bridge and my father would lift me up and sit me right on the edge with my legs dangling over the water far below. He would then just stare at me and ask me how the water made me feel. My mum started to get worried about these daily walks and asked me where we went, when I told her what we did and what my father used to say to me she went white. She wasted no more time and after yet another visit from our doctor my dad was taken into hospital. We later learned from a doctor that my dad had wanted to commit suicide by throwing himself off of a bridge and he had only taken me with him to stop himself from doing it, he said I could never have done it with Susan with me. To my young mind he seemed to be in and out of Hospital for years and it was a life we just had to get used to, but it never got any easier.

On one of our visits to him he surprised us by meeting us at the hospital station, he got hold of mum's arm and said, start walking, either I'm coming home with you or I'm going to throw us all under the next train, mum walked with him and was nearly fainting away because she was holding my brother in her arms at the time, John was about two and a half years old by then. All poor mum could do was get on the train with us again and pray. Once we arrived back home, unknown to my father the Police, doctors and straight jacket were waiting and the terrible cycle started all over again.

The time that stands out in my mind as being the scariest experience of all was when my brother was about 3 years old. Dad was again very mentally sick and had been so for a few months, he was laid in the front room on a mattress saying he had cancer, and he was convinced he was going to die. He would only eat some cornflakes once a day and mum was at her wits end. She contacted Dr Radcliff and he came to visit us. It was a job to get anyone up the stairs because dad would not allow it, but on this occasion he agreed. Dr Radcliff saw the state my father was in and how much weight he had lost (he was like a skeleton). He said "ok Harry, what's up then?" My dad told him that he had cancer, but then added that he wasn't going into hospital. Dr Radcliff agreed with him and said he would get him some medicine. Out of earshot he pulled my mum to one side and told her he would arrange for an ambulance and police to come and take my very sick father away. Mum was petrified and so was I. The next thing I knew the police were creeping up the stairs along with the medics. Somehow dad knew something was happening he seemed to have a sixth sense, he grabbed John and ran to the window, mum screamed and then the police and medics ran up the stairs and came bursting into the room, mum by now was fainting away. The police made a grab for my brother and caught him just in time, then fought to restrain my dad. He was then straight jacketed and taken away. I remember feeling very sad and frightened, but happy that my brother was safe.

It was not only the fear and hardship caused by my father's illness which caused us pain, sometimes the people around us made a bad situation worse. One day when my father was yet again away from us in hospital knocks went at our door and mum looked out over the balcony to see who it was, she saw one of my dad's brothers (Johnny) who was godfather to my little brother, he was also a very wealthy man (as many of our relations seemed to be). Johnny began to rant and shouted up to my mother that she was the cause of Harry's illness; mum could not believe it and was so upset that she had been turned on like this. It seemed clear to us that none of my father's family ever accepted his mental illness, it was too much of a stigma for them to handle so they needed a scapegoat. Poor mum I don't know how she ever coped with all the stress which came our way, we always seemed to be alone and if not for auntie Amy (who was not even family) we really would have been.

Everybody else was afraid of coming to see us, out of fear or shame, it didn't matter which, we were still alone. Before my fathers illness I remember that every Sunday evening, Uncle Len, Uncle Ern and dad's friend from the railway Harry Marsham would come round to our house and mum would prepare sandwiches while they all played cards and had fun with my dad. It's funny because when he came home that first time after his illness, no one came round. Only uncle Ern would show his face occasionally, my father lost all of his so called friends. As I got older I realised mum was on her own and needed help so I used to look after John while mum went on her cleaning jobs, I became very responsible, like a little mum myself, doing housework and all sorts, but I never minded at all, it was my family.

Old Enough To Know

Like Sue I was growing up now and was old enough to know that my dad had been sick, We all used to visit him in Cain Hill and I too can vividly remember the train journey and then bus trip up that long steep hill and even that terrible hospital smell when we finally arrived, but most of all I remember hoping that the next time he came home my dad would be well.

At that time we all slept in one big bed in our damp back bedroom, which meant we could help keep each other warm on cold nights. It is hard to believe by today's standards but not only didn't we have a kitchen (we had a small landing with an old gas cooker) we also only had one little tiny sink with a single cold tap which was placed down one flight of stairs from the landing. To us it was normal to have an all over wash in a bowl in front of the fire, which was the closest we could come to having a bath, and to heat all of our water in a kettle because our sink never had a hot tap. Years later when the sink was finally replaced we found out that it had originally been for emptying and cleaning out old Victorian bed pans (or piss pots as the cockneys called them) but we knew no better then so maybe what you never have you never miss?

When my dad did eventually come back to us as he had done before, it seemed that maybe this time the combination of terrible shock treatment and medication had finally worked, but with so many people attaching the stigma of nutcase and madman to him it was hard for my family to get back to any thing resembling a normal life. Time passed and we struggled on and by then some of mums sisters had begun to visit us again and did their best to help us out, (better late than never). Our Aunt Eady was a God send to us during those early desperate times and every Christmas she would get a Provident cheque and take my mum, my sister and I to buy food and clothing which at least gave us some hope during what was supposed to be the festive season. Eventually my dad got a job with a firm as a van driver, and with his medication working things at last seemed to be looking brighter, we had got our dad back and Maggie had at last got her Harry back, but little did she know that when he came home he was always destined to bring the other side of Harry with him.

We never really knew just what triggered my father's illness but something we later heard could have had something to do with it. When he was a young boy Harry had fallen off of his bike and hit his head, he was knocked unconscious and remained that way for two days. No one took him to hospital and all his mother did was wrap his head in vinegar and brown paper (like the old nursery rhyme) and put him in a dark room till he woke up. Who knows just what damage could have been done then, you never know?

It Never Rains But It Pours

Our problems were not only centred around my fathers illness. As I began to grow up a little I would often start to cry at night and say my legs hurt, well after a while mum realised something was wrong so she took me to the doctors who then sent me to Great Ormond street hospital for children, it was there that it was found that my knees were growing inward and down, and if not corrected I would have a major problem in later life, I would even have trouble walking.   I was tested and measured many times and for the next three years I had to wear special built up shoes, not quite Frankenstein shoes, but to my little legs they felt that way, but thanks to the wonderful Hospital who's patron is Peter Pan, the shoes worked, and when I think of all the things I am able to do today it seems like a miracle, maybe they should call me Forest Gump Carrigan.

Adding more pain to her life, as if my lovely mum did not already have enough to deal with, she started to suffer from burning chest pains and would vomit up acid after meals, which meant weight started to fall off her already slim figure. Mum was sent to the hospital who diagnosed a hiatus hernia, which would be difficult to correct without major surgery, so she was forced to be on medication for the rest of her life and was never truly rid of the symptoms, but as always she never complained, she just accepted it as part of her life and got on with it.   I hated seeing mum rubbing her chest with pain night after night, or being out with her and seeing her suddenly have to vomit acid up into a hanky, if it sounds horrible to read imagine how it must have felt coping with it on top of all the other trauma in her life. I am thankful to say that in later years the plastic kind of tablets she used to take along with her medicine seemed to seal her hernia and make it so much more manageable for her, but it never completely went away.

There were also quite a few times when mum caught pleurisy due to the often freezing conditions she was forced to work in. One time she contracted this illness while working at night on Waterloo station and she became really ill. She was signed off from work by our long time family doctor (Dr Radcliff) and my sister had to go to the chemist to collect her medication. Mum was prescribed antibiotics and stuff called Thermogine wool which Sue then helped wrap around her chest to keep the heat in, but instead of going to bed as the doctor had ordered, mum went right back out to work telling my sister through tears of despair and pain, I can't afford not to work.

More Family

Time went by and our early childhood started to have some happy times, one day my sister befriended a stray dog she had found, it was a black and white cross collie someone must have abandoned, we all fell in love with her and called her Suzy, our new family member. My auntie Vi had done well with her life and married a shop owner (Jim) so compared to us Aunt Vi and uncle Jim were very rich. My mum and her sister were close and as I said earlier in the book mum used to clean her house for extra money, when she did this I used to go with her and marvelled at my Aunt's magic home with hot water and its own toilet and bath (wow).

For one of my birthdays Aunt Vi bought me a little Yorkshire terrier and we called her Foo Foo. Foo Foo was not a tiny weedy little dog with a ribbon, although we tried to put one on her head a couple of times, but it lasted only minutes before it was shaken off and chewed up. Suzy met Foo and became friends for life, we also had fish in a big tank, two rabbits which we kept on the rooftop veranda (which for some reason we called the lids?) and a budgie called Joey. We had a lot of love to give and gave it to each other and our animals freely.

We had been brought up in an atmosphere of giving, sharing and caring in spite of what we were going through. I can remember being at school and a teacher holding up nine sweets and saying to us, "I want to give you all a sweet but we do not have enough to go around" (we had ten in our little class) "who is willing to give up their sweet so our new classmate Linda can have one". No one seemed willing to do this so I stuck up my little hand right away and volunteered to give away my sweet. With this selfless act the teacher said, "Because John was willing to go without for someone else, he can now have two sweets". Our teacher had plenty of sweets hidden away; it was just a test and a lesson. This kind of attitude came directly from mum and dad and sometimes this, let me help attitude backfired.

I don't remember how we came to meet them but a family latched on to us and we opened our home to them. They seemed to have even less than us, including nowhere to live. The memory is foggy now but I know that it ended up with us going away hop picking and coming home to find that they had stolen what little we had left behind in Oswin Street, they also abandoned their Alsatian dog who would not let us back in our front room. It took big Amy from next door who threw a whole bucket of water over the crazed animal, driving it out so it could be caught and taken away. But that was not the end of it, the Police turned up at our house not long after and said that this family had been going all over the country as the Carrigans and committing fraud where ever they went. Luckily because of my fathers past we had no trouble convincing them that it was not us.

Another time we extended the hand of friendship ended up being much more rewarding but with a tinge of sadness at the same time. One night we were sleeping in the old hopping huts during one of our yearly trips when a loud knocking was heard at our large barn like front door, which my dad had created for extra safety. When we warily opened it we saw the local Police man accompanied by some other strangers all with torches in their hands. When they saw my parents they apologised and said they were looking for two runaways from a Borstal (a kind of juvenile home for troublesome boys) and after seeing the light in the huts they thought it might be them. When they left we all had trouble getting over the shock and going back to sleep. In the morning we were all up bright and early ready to continue with our yearly adventure and noticed that one of the old derelict brick hopping huts which no one had used for years had been opened. When we looked inside we found two young lads in their early teens who looked as shocked to see us as we were to see them. When mum and dad had made sure they were no threat to us we got speaking to them, and they told us that they had no parents and had got into some trouble which had meant them ending up in Borstal. They begged my mum and dad not to turn them in and to let them stay a while in the old huts. It ended up with my mum feeding them and looking after them for a few days and they got on well with us, I think they just tolerated the little boy full of questions and probably liked my sister more than me. They were very well mannered to us all and it was quite sad when the police and the men from the home turned up again to take them away.

When we eventually returned home to London we received a letter from the boys asking if my parents would adopt them, it was all so sad. With my poor dad the way he was, all my mum could say was a regretful no. We never knew what happened to the boys but one of them had a saying which was, you're not bad for your age on a Wednesday, which my sister and I still say to each other even today, which I suppose is our way of never forgetting the boys who wanted to become part of our family. Whether it was stray people or stray animals my family would always be there for them, and I still do that job today whenever I can.

The Darling Buds

As I said earlier in this book many old London families took their holidays each year fruit and hop picking in Kent, well we came from one of those families and for generations it was the only holiday the Healys and the Carrigans ever had. Each year in June we would get so excited because we knew it was time to travel a million miles at least (or so it felt) and go to Kent. We became famous in our street because everyone knew that in the summer the Carrigan family would hire a big furniture van and load up all but the kitchen sink (including all the animals, fish tank and all) and go off for their four month adventure.

Because of the situation with my father's and now my mother's health, the education authorities allowed my sister and I to have months of school work to take with us (which we had to do) and my family were seen as a special case for convalescent holidays. We all went to a village in Kent called Plaxtol where my mum's mum had gone before her, we would clean out the old hopper hut's (as people called them) and furnish them with all the comforts of home, well nearly all. The huts were in a special little valley between the woods and the hop field on Cannons farm, it really seemed like a paradise to us. In the early years lots of members of both my father and mother's families would all go fruit and hop picking and every hut would be filled with either friends or relations, but in the end it was only us left. On the site there was only one fresh water tap and an open fronted cook house with a big open fire which was our only means of cooking, but we loved it.

During those months my family would earn enough money to help see us through the winter, with dad driving tractors, bailing hay, and then picking fruit with the rest of us. Harry was also the entertainment in the local village pub (The Papermakers Arms) on his piano every weekend, and the whole village would wait for our return year after year to join in with the old London sing alongs which dad would be requested to play. The Papermakers was a lovely old family pub which had a small walled off snug bar where they would allow children to be, this was the place I would sit with my mum and some of her fruit picking friends and sometimes I would stand on a chair to look over the bar at all the happy goings on and watch my dad on the piano. I do not know how it began but it came to be that during one year I became the star turn with my dad on a Saturday evening. I would proudly march into the main bar to sing on the mike, and then proceed to bring the house down with my rendition of the dance called the twist. They really were the happiest time of our lives and the only place on Earth my mum ever really wanted to end up.

There used to be a TV series called The Darling Buds Of May and my memories of those days really were like that series, full of sunshine green fields and happiness, I remember spending hours battling hoards of stinging nettles with a stick, because I was really a knight in armour and they were armies of bad Trolls, even then I wanted to be the hero.

The story of the Londoners coming down to Kent to pick hops is now almost like a lost legend, and it is hard to believe it ever really happened or that I was really a part of it. In the old hopping days some of the men would get long wooden poles with a hook on the end and pull the rough hop vines down from where they hung, then take them over to the hop bins (as they were called). The women and children would then strip the hops off of the vines and into sacks. This would leave the hop pickers hands literally hop green and smelling of the pungent hops for days to come. I was just young enough to remember the last days of hopping before technology caught up and hop machines took over, bringing the demise of a whole way of life.

As I have said with the end of hopping all the other families from London ceased to make their yearly pilgrimage, all but the Carrigans that is. We still made our trip to the Cannons farm from June through to September, to begin our fruit picking holiday (which was so much more to us). We started with strawberries then moved on to raspberries, black currents, gooseberries, cherries, plums and finally apples. During our many trips through out the years, the older I became the more time I would spend picking fruit and the less time I would spend playing. Eventually I grew responsible enough and strong enough to join mum and dad picking cherries, plums and apples up in the trees, I also learned the way to carry the heavy tall ladders and balance them to the sky as we walked through the orchards. When we picked the apples we had large bags strapped to our backs, which would get really heavy and awkward when full of apples, especially when you were at the top of a ladder high in a tree, and when you took them off at the end of the day you would feel like you were walking in zero gravity and almost floated home.

On one occasion mum was high up a ladder and leaned to pick an apple, as she did the apples in her bag shifted to one side which made her ladder twist in the tree. This sent mum crashing down through the middle of the tree and she was only saved when her legs caught on two branches which had crossed about ten feet off the ground. On hearing mums cries we all ran over to find her hanging upside down, shocked but thankfully unharmed. If I had a time machine those are the days I would re-visit, The Darling Buds of May.

Violence Rears It's Ugly Head

My father's illness went in cycles, from periods of normality to ever increasing symptoms of insanity, after that first devastating attack on my mum and dad's up and down slow recovery, the illness returned like waves on a sea shore but was then absent for a long period of time and we dared to hope. But as they say, the only sure thing is change.

It was the swinging sixties, the Beatles, mini skirts and … Schizophrenia. Harry's moods were ever changing, and he began to say strange things. At one time he even said that his real name was Darmen Christianson! Sometimes he would even use a strange voice. He started to say our house was bugged, and would jump up and take all the light bulbs out of their sockets, which meant we would all sit for hours in darkness, and one time for some reason he painted all the glass lampshades and bulbs in our house red, which made it look like some kind of brothel. But a worse change started to happen, he turned violent.

Harry began to accuse my sister of lying to him, and said that (THEY) had been getting to her (the word "they" would crop up a lot). We now had the top four rooms in 27 Oswin Street and Sue had her own room. In one fit of rage dad tore down all of the pop posters Sue had pinned on her walls which she had painstakingly cut from magazines, and then pulled her across the floor by her long hair. The violence toward Sue also moved onto him physically slapping her around the face and going for her so strongly that she would hide underneath our dining room table to escape his rage. Many times to prevent himself from turning on his family, my father would drive our dog Suzy under the sideboard by kicking her terribly, her yelps of pain still echo in my mind today. Mum would try to prevent these attacks on my sister and our dog but that only made him turn his attention to her, not with physical violence but always with the threat of it.

One frightening event which stands out in my mind began one tea time. We used to have a high cupboard with a fold down front flap which we used to prepare our food on (tea etc) the doors of this unit had big glass oval shapes in and I can remember my father sitting in the armchair while mum prepared food at the cupboard. Harry suddenly started to accuse my mum of getting secret messages from the TV about him and wanting him put away, mum said "don't be silly Harry" and gave a small cough, my dad jumped up and said her cough was another secret message, then without warning he punched just past mum's face and through the glass on the door, as we all froze in shock he put his face next to mum's and said in a voice like something from the Exorcist, if my hand is cut when I pull it out, you are next, thankfully and miraculously it was not.

The only time my father ever touched me with anything remotely like violence was one Sunday, again in the bad sixties. Almost every Sunday one of my mum's sisters Emily (Em for short) would come to see us with her daughter Genie and Aunt Em would always bring prawns or crab sticks, usually some kind of sea food we could never afford. This Sunday started off in a good atmosphere, with dad playfully fighting with mum, she was making out she was a boxer and everyone was laughing, until the other side of Harry suddenly stepped forward. Dad's face changed and he grabbed mum by her ankles, picked her up and with strength born of insanity began to swing her round the room with her head narrowly missing the furniture and my Aunt. Even at my young age I knew something was wrong and I had to do something so as he spun I jumped on my Dad's back from off of the sofa, the next I knew I had been shrugged off across the room crashing onto the floor, Dad dropped mum and shouted for my Aunt to get out, which she did very quickly, Harry controlled himself but still had a crazed look on his face and he demanded that I be put to bed right away. My mum still very shaken from what she had been through took me to the bedroom and locked us in, this happened on a Sunday afternoon and we came out of the bedroom on Monday tea time. When we eventually surfaced my dad could not apologise enough and seemed really upset that he had touched me, by this time he had again returned to being the loving Harry and we could again relax, almost.

The only other time my Father directed anything at me which resembled aggression was again when I was quite young. I was outside in the street playing cowboys and Indians with my friends and I had a lovely little cowboy suit on which I had got for Christmas. I saw my dad walking down the road coming back from one of his daily walks, so I ran up to him with my little cowboy gun and went bang. With that he grabbed me by the arm and dragged me into the house and up the stairs shouting, I won't let them turn you into one of them (I was frightened stiff), he shouted for my mum who came running and he made her take the outfit off of me and put me in bed for the rest of the day. I was in tears and just could not understand what I had done to upset my dad. Mum stayed with me to ease my tears as always, but I never forgot that day. During his bad times he always hated the Americans and would often bring mum to tears by shouting that she wanted to run off with some big Yank, so I can only suppose that my little cowboy suit had somehow sent him over the edge that day. Who knows?

My dad used to love football and when I was about eleven or twelve he began to take me and all my mates every Sunday to the local aptly named, Bedlam Park for football practice. We would all have a great game of football and dad would join in as well as coach us, we even talked about creating a real local football team with Harry as our coach. One Sunday towards the end of the year we were all involved in our great Sunday match when my friend Kevin kicked the ball right into Harry's face (and Kevin could kick like a mule) my dad staggered about for a second holding his face then rushed after the ball which had gone back into play, he then proceeded to charge into every one of us with the look of possession on his face and one by one knocked us all to the floor (even me). When he had decimated all of us he just turned and barked, we are going home. That incident ended our Sunday football outings and my friends never dared to come out with us again.

The Harry We Loved

At this point I feel I need to speak out in defence of my father, because when the illness was not on him he was really a fantastic person. First of all he was honest to a fault and really belonged in the Knights of armour days, he always spoke of honour and truth, and about always doing the right thing, he would take me and many of the children from our street on day trips and look after us like a hawk, and I remember many happy trips to the zoo to see the animals. He would always be immaculately dressed and clean, and on most days if he was going outside he would wear a suit and tie. He always carried his trusted umbrella with him and in fact he looked very much like John Steed from the old Avengers TV show.

My dad liked to read a lot and was for all he had been through quite a cultured man, he was a great pianist, singer and song writer and in fact had fate not dealt him that hand I am sure he would have made a great success of his life, as did all of his brothers who ended up very well off. My father was a lovely kind man with a wonderful sense of fun and humour when his illness let him, which was most of the time. But we always waited for the storm so it was hard to enjoy the sun. One thing my dad did seem to possess was a gift for healing, where this came from we never knew.

The first time I remember it showing itself was when a young girl fell over and badly gashed her knee during the hopping days, it looked terrible and really needed stitches, my dad held her wound closed, dried the surrounding area and pulled a plaster tightly across the gaping cut so she could be taken to hospital, when they got her there the doctor who dealt with the situation said, the wound has closed and needs no stitches, whoever put the dressing on must have a background in medicine. Well my dad had spent a long time in hospitals but not for learning purposes. He also helped me more than once.

I had run through some brambles and tore the back of my legs when I was younger and along the scars had grown about a hundred tiny warts, I also had a really big wart on my knee which no amount of treatment had been able to get rid of. One day my father took a look at my wart covered leg and just said I am going to rub a big old Spanish onion over your warts for a couple of days, then they will fall off? We did not believe for a moment they would but we humoured Harry (as we so often did) and after three days I woke up to find my bed full of warts, every last one had fallen off, (they never came back). I also suffered from chronic hay fever for years which dad again cured, one day he made me sniff up a load of pepper, so I sneezed and sneezed till I could sneeze no more, My hay fever vanished never to return, He also saved mum from an operation, she had grown a lump on the lid of her eye which the doctor had diagnosed as a cyst, he said she would need surgery to remove it, well the night before she was due to have it done my dad said come over here a moment Maggie, he had a bowel of hot water and a handkerchief ready, he bathed her eye for what must have been half an hour then began to work over her eye with the hanky, all of a sudden he said, all done and in the hanky was a large grey stone which he had removed from her eye, when she went to the Hospital the next morning they sent her straight home again, the cyst was gone. The last thing he helped me with could have been really bad if not for him.

I was about ten years of age and was eager to run down stairs to play with my friends but I needed to go to the toilet for a pee. I was in such a rush that as I left the toilet and zipped up my fly I caught my little manhood right in the zip pull its self. I screamed out and dad came running down the stairs, I was bent double and in agony, he carried me upstairs and calmed me down, then with mum standing by proceeded to go to work on me. I was well and truly threaded right through the zip and the zip pull with no way out, well doctor Harry first got a razor blade and cut my trousers and pants off of me, then spent two hours with a pair of pliers clipping minute bits of metal from my trapped little…thing. He had sweat running down his face (so did I), well he freed me and without so much as a scar. He did seem to have some kind of gift for healing; perhaps it was to balance up his other tortured side. Who knows what he would have become without his illness, maybe even a doctor himself?

I have a little notebook which my father carried everywhere, and in it he wrote lyrics for songs and little sayings which meant something to him. On one page he has nothing but these few words written large in pencil. **Her Smile Is Lovely, But Oh How Wonderful Her Grin.** I am sure he wrote that about my mother. He never showed anyone his book so he must have written it just for himself. This shows a little of the real other side of Harry, the man he would have always been, but for that cursed illness.

Betraying The Trust

When my dad began to get ill again mum would secretly go to our doctor to tell him, but the hardest part of all this was the fact that none of us could ever let my father know we thought he was ill, to him the rest of the world was against him and we were the only ones on his side that he could trust, so we could never be seen as the ones who were betraying him, for reasons of love and safety. I have a vivid memory of mum saying, come with me love, and leading me out of our front room with tears streaming down her face which she dare not let my dad see, going down the stairs as six men passed us on the way up, hearing raised voices and then the screams of my father shouting "NO NO", and then calling out "MAGGIE MAGGIE", then terrible noises of fighting, crashes, screams, then the sight of my dad being carried out of the house in a straight jacket with the neighbours looking on. Our poor father was to go away to mental hospitals no less that eleven times in his life, sometimes raging and fighting, sometimes voluntarily.

One of those times which could again so easily have ended in tragedy was in the early part of dad's illness during the sixties, he was displaying signs of increasing paranoia and mum began to get worried, so she once more contacted the doctors, obviously someone un familiar with my fathers case took charge this time because a lone doctor arrived at our house and told my mum that he wanted to talk to Harry himself before deciding on any action. My mother made him give his word that he would not let Harry know who had sent for him and he agreed, well almost the first words from this so called intelligent doctor's mouth were. So Mr Carrigan your wife tells us that you are feeling unwell again…You can imagine how those words cut into mum like a knife and made her blood run cold, the doctor then ordered her out of the room. After an hour or so the doctor emerged and with a steely stare said to my mum, that man is as sane as Jesus Christ, no treatment is necessary, maybe you could do with some counselling yourself. As I said before my dad was a very intelligent man and had obviously worked out just what he needed to say to convince this doctor that he was completely sane, he must have put on a great act. My poor mum pleaded with the doctor not to go without taking Harry with him and said you can't leave me alone with him after he knows I sent for you. The doctor said she was over reacting and left. As soon as he was gone my dad barricaded himself and my mum in the front room, dragged her to the balcony and threatened to throw them both off. Thus began a Police siege which could have ended in disaster, but thank God it ended with my dad giving himself up and going away yet again to that hospital on the hill.

Up The Hill

My life as a young child is full of memories of long train journeys to someplace where a special Bus would meet us then take us up a long tree lined hill to a massive castle like building, this I later learned was the infamous Cain Hill mental asylum where my dad spent many long visits, he also frequented a few other mental establishments during the years to come, all as daunting as each other but none as daunting as Cain Hill. I can remember running up a long corridor which had a large white metal door at the end with a small square sliding hatch, my mum would lift me up to press a large golden button on the wall which made a loud buzzing sound, the hatch would slide back and I would say, I am here to see my daddy Harry. Once inside that door I can remember thinking, why do all these people look so strange and move so slowly, and I always hated that hospital smell which seemed to stay with us even after we left.

As I grew older I used to hear kids at school argue, and one would say to the other, you're a Cain Hill nutter you are, which when I was old enough to understand really hurt me inside, and even though it was not directed at me, in a way it always would be.

There was one time when the doctors again almost cost my mother dear. On one occasion during a bout of my dad's illness, for some reason his paranoia convinced him that it was my mum who had Schizophrenia, this got so bad that he insisted on taking HER to a general hospital. When they arrived he told doctors it was a sad case and that she would never admit to being ill, also that she might try to harm herself. When the doctors were at last alone with mum she of course said to them that it was Harry who was ill, but like some kind of nightmare they would not believe her, they even took all her sharp objects and matches away from her, at one point seeing my mothers obvious agitation they even wanted to give her a sedative, and were about to when someone found all of Harry's past records. The doctors could not apologise enough.

The Not So Swinging Sixties

My fathers schizophrenia first surfaced during the late 1950s and went through many phases and states, from violent to religious, to persecution to hypochondria and the ever constant secret organisation complex (or them), and as I have touched on before in this book, in the Sixties it seemed that he went through them all, one after another. But In between the bad times during the Sixties and early Seventies we did have some good normal times when Harry was his real lovely self, and we were thankful for that, but they were all too few and far between.

One of my sisters friends (Linda Bailey) used to come round to our house and often used to hear dad playing on his beloved piano which he had done for years, (it was his only real hobby and passion) sometimes Linda would go into dad's piano room with him and end up having a sing along, Linda wanted to one day be a singer and had a good voice to go with her ambition, so dad began to write a song a for her called "I don't want to know anything about you", and when it was finished she could really belt it out and sang it very well. They started to rehearse together and it was decided that Harry would be her manager in her bid for stardom, but alas as with most of the good things in dad's life his constant relapses into the dreaded illness got in the way and shattered more dreams, Linda never became a singer. Harry did continue with his song writing though and at one point he even dropped off some music at the Beatles Apple company, never to be heard of again.

At the height of his paranoia Harry would sit with a hanky pressed to his face convinced that someone was behind our gas fire in the chimney blowing out poison gas and smoke into our front room, this sounds so ludicrous to me now as to be almost funny, but it was all part of the torture he went through which he in turn then passed on to us. If it was not the poison gas then the TV would be bugged or "they" were watching us through it. If not that then all the light bulbs were microphones and had to be taken out plunging us into darkness. At one time it really did seem never ending.

To bring to a close what really were the dreaded sixties for us I really must cover a couple more instances which led to my dad being hospitalised yet again. One day he was acting very agitated and said he wanted to take me out for a walk (I must have been about eight years of age) mum would not allow this so she tried to humour him by saying, that would be nice Harry I will come with you, as mum went to put on her coat dad said to me lets play a game, we are going to run and mum will try and catch us, with that he grabbed my hand and we ran down the stairs and up the street, just as we turned the corner of our road a number twelve bus was just about to pull away, so I was lifted still running on to the bus. As it pulled away I remember seeing my mum run around the corner frantically looking for me, but having no idea I was on the bus, I now know that my panic struck mum rang the police right away and an all points went out to look for us. We spent the day over the West end of London and also visited all the major parks, Harry brought me home just as it was getting dark with no help from the police. Soon after this episode Harry started to say he was being poisoned so he stopped eating and would only drink water. The weight just fell off of him and his life really was in danger so he had to go away yet again to prevent him starving to death.

The reason for my father's schizophrenia being under control for a while and breaking out again and again was that when he was at his worst my father was given the horrible but necessary electric shock treatment which does work for the short term, and when my dad used to come home from hospital he would be on medication, and that worked until he started flushing his tablets down the toilet, which would invariably let the genie out of the bottle again. The only alternative was to keep dad in a mental hospital for the rest of his life, which (if you had seen the inside of those places in those days) would have been a terrible fate to consign my father to. I know that in her heart my lovely loyal mum always believed that one day the Harry she married, the Harry she loved would return for good. As they say, hope springs eternal.

Money Matters

During all the years of mayhem following my father's breakdown money had been tight to say the least, with Harry constantly going away, losing his job, coming out and trying for work again, it meant frequent visits for my mum to what she used to call the UAB, to sit in front of unsympathetic people who would decide how much money we could have to help us survive these desperate times.

The last full time job my dad had was for a delivery firm, which he really enjoyed doing, I remember sometimes being allowed to go with him for the day and seeing all manor of brown paper parcels piled up in the back of his van. He held this job for quite a long time, he was well and things were looking up. One day he was at his depot and had a large carpet across his shoulder which weighed quite a bit, as he walked across the yard a piece of cardboard was covering a hole in the ground and as my father stepped on it his foot went into the hole and with all of the weight of the carpet, his ankle snapped as it twisted under him, the pain must have been sickening. In today's world I am sure that he could have made a claim for some kind of compensation, but then no one was in his corner to advise him. It was months before he could walk again and left him with years of problems and pain from that ankle, thus ended my dad's real working life. He did many jobs on the farm in Kent over the years and even helped out family members when they offered him a days work in their shops or pubs or businesses, but apart from long months on the farm over the years the rest only amounted to a few days at best. Someone amongst all our so called family members could have offered him a helping hand; he was never lazy, just ill.

All of this meant that through out all the years of trouble it was up to my poor mum to try and provide for our family, alone. My sister Sue told me that there was a time when mum couldn't even afford a new pair of boots. The boots she used to wear were the kind with zips at the front and went up to the ankle, not because they were in fashion but because they were warm during the many cold conditions she worked in. Before she started work she would cut out a large piece of cardboard and put it in the bottom of her boots to cover the holes which had worn in the soles. It really was that bad at times.

Mum often said that one of the worst feelings in the world is to feel obligated and I later found out that she had always borrowed to help us get by, either from relations or money lenders and many years later she said that she always felt that she was forced to go through life owing people, if not money then favours and they had never let her forget it. Mum at one time used to clean our Aunt Vi and uncle Jims flat for £1.00 a week and she would walk to the flat at the far end of London's East Lane in all weathers because she could not afford the bus fare. My Aunt would also often lend money to mum (her sister) to buy us kids some clothes, but mum always paid her every penny back. My sister told me that she had always thought our Aunt had given her money as a gift to help us until one day she found mums pay back book.

My mother was also sometimes seen as an easy touch because she was so hard working and desperate for money. One time she had an early morning cleaning job to clean offices near Lambeth Bridge and left my sister to look after me at 4.30 am, saying she would be home by 7. She had begun the job ok but it seemed that every day she was given more and more offices to clean, until one day she noticed there did not seem to be any other cleaners about! Mum went searching through the building and found that all the other cleaners including the charge hand were asleep in an office and mum had been fooled into doing their work. Needless to say she left that job but not before making it clear just what she thought of her co-workers. Mum arrived home crying and exhausted after that experience. That's why mum hated the obligation she was forced to feel most of her life.

Beauty And The Little Beast

One bright moment around those times involved my sister Susan. As she was growing up Sue had been spending more and more time at my Aunt Vi's house, Aunt Vi and uncle Jim now owned a chain of grocery stores around the area and lived above one in the famous Lambeth Walk, it was a way for Sue to have some normality in her life, Aunt Vi also gave her a job as a Saturday girl in the Lambeth Walk shop, which later turned into a full time job. Susan was now sixteen and had turned into a very beautiful looking girl so my Aunt entered her in a big beauty contest. My dad was very protective of Sue and me, sometimes in a rational way and sometimes not, so no one told him about the contest until it was over. Low and behold, Sue won the contest and the title of Miss Lambeth Walk which culminated in a large parade through the streets with my sister perched on top of an open limousine with tickertape, cameras and crowds everywhere.

As the parade drove down the Lambeth Walk I was in the crowd with my mum waving and shouting with the rest, it was plain to see by looking at mum's face how proud she felt that Sue could have won the contest after all she had been through during her early years. Looking back on it, it was quite an achievement. As Sue drove by, a large woman standing beside us said out loud, I think she is fucking ugly, why did they pick her I bet she won it on her back. I saw my mum's face turn to thunder, then snap back enjoying the proud moment.

Later that day after all the excitement and the crowds had gone mum and I were walking home. As we passed a house mum stopped and said to me, just wait here a minute love, she then marched up the path to the front door of the house and knocked, the door opened and I saw the mountain of a woman, it was the one who had thrown insults at my sister during the parade. It was obvious that they knew each other as my little mum and the mountain exchanged some heated words, the next second my mum literally jumped up at the woman and punched her full in the face, she staggered back into her house and disappeared from view, without a word mum marched back down the path took my hand, "said come on boy", and we toddled off home. Mum was only a small woman but her heart was as big as the great out doors and she would do anything to protect or stick up for her kids.

I got on quite well with my sister but I did drive her mad at times. As an off shoot of her winning the beauty contest Sue was offered some modelling work. Well I took it upon myself to embark on a reign of practical jokes, which to Sue at that time must have been anything but funny; it really was the beauty and the little beast. One day she was getting ready to go on a modelling assignment and as she was about to leave I pinned a sheet of newspaper across the top of her half open bedroom door and poured a bag of white flour on top of the paper, well you can guess what happened next, as Sue came out looking perfect after hours of getting ready and walked through the doorway the paper tore and she was covered in flour (I am cringing as I write this). As you might guess and fully understand Sue exploded and mum had to stop her from killing me (which I would have deserved). I also used to stick signs on her back just before she left the house saying all sorts of silly things, and one day she was given a really expensive wig for a shoot so I proceeded to give it a hair cut. All horrible stuff really, but I was only being the little brother-a pain in the arse. We did have some fun together though too.

My dad's mother lived by herself on the second floor of 27 Oswin Street. She was about four foot nothing in height but boy, was she full of spite or what. She would accuse Sue of being (as she put it) a tart, and would say that I used to pee up the wall in the toilet? She also said our dog's (Suzy and Foo) used to crap on her floor, well we actually caught her splashing water from a kettle up the wall of the toilet, and also dropping bits of pooh she had picked up from the street in a little coal shovel, all of which she denied, well we wanted revenge.

One night I cut a giant moth shape out of a cabbage leaf and dangled it over the banister outside of her room, as she came out into the dim light the green monster moth touched her face and she started to scream and shout for my dad's brother Bobby, who lived downstairs. Now Bobby wore glasses as thick as milk bottles but this night he ran up the stairs without them on, he grabbed a broom and shouted get behind me mother I'll get it, as he proceeded to go to battle with the deadly cabbage moth. Upstairs my sister and I were nearly peeing ourselves with laughter.

A few years later my Nan accused me of having orgies in my room, (chance would be a fine thing) believe me with my up bringing under the eyes of good old Harry boy I did not have a clue what to do with a girl let alone have an orgy, so it was time for more revenge.

My Nan was from an age where snuff taking was all the rage, and she still indulged in this horrible habit, she would open her little silver snuff tin and with her long fingers take a big pinch of this horrible brown powder, put it up to her nose and take a big sniff. Well this sparked off an idea in me, so one day after she had toddled off to the betting shop (she loved horse racing, so did my dad) I went into her room, tipped away all of her snuff from its tin and replaced it with drinking chocolate powder. Later that night I went down to take her a newspaper and at that moment she was opening her prised silver snuff tin (I just had to see this) as I stood talking and trying to keep a straight face, she took a big pinch and sniffed, as she carried on talking to me a horrible brown trickle started to come down from her nose toward her mouth, I said bye Nan and quickly turned to go so she did not see my ear to ear grin, as I went I started to sing, hot chocolate drinking chocolate hot chocolate etc, she never knew.

Then There Were Three

My sister was trying to make a career out of modelling while still working in my Aunt's shop, it was also the time in her life when boyfriends were on the scene, Harry was still going up and down with his state of mind and Sue needed her freedom.

Aunt Vi agreed to let Sue move in with her and Uncle Jim, they had plenty of room and although I am sure my dad was not really happy about it he agreed to let Sue go. So it was that Sue's shot at a normal life began. As time went on we began to see less and less of Sue and in the end who could really blame her. I do not really know just what my sister got up to during those early years of her new found freedom, but I think Sue embraced her new life and made up for all the years under my father's gaze.

This is where I begin to tell the rest of the story through my eyes, about my life, because now it was just my mum and I who would have to face the other side of Harry. There are many memories from those early times after Sue departed, but one thing which stays with me and reflects the tone of those dark years.

I still have a vivid a memory of my mum and I sitting in the dark on our small landing with only the blue glow of the gas flames flickering over us from the open oven door which we were huddled around. This scene happened quite a few times in my young life, mum and I sitting together, sometimes on a cold winter's night after my dad had removed all the light bulbs from our home because he thought they were bugged, or after one of the London blackouts which plagued Britain during those days of the miners strikes. But the lasting memory is of mum, always telling me that the hard life we had, would not last forever, always trying to keep me positive, knowing that even at my young age what effect this kind of occurrence could have on me, so she made sure it was never a frightening time, she made it almost as if we were around a camp fire. The only time those dark cold nights had any fear attached to them was when we heard the door knob being turned beside us, as Harry emerged from the darkness of the front room, the fear was, not knowing which Harry would be in the doorway. Even now when I check the oven to see how the Sunday roast is doing and I see those blue flames, I am taken back to my lovely mum who never let us give in to the darkness.

Pain In The Rain

There are moments and things in your life that stand out as defining events, this is one of them.

I am not sure of my age or just when in our lives this happened, but I do remember I was young and had been playing in the street outside our house with my friends Debbie and Kevin, as we played the heavens suddenly opened and rain began to pour down, we didn't let a little thing like rain stop us so we carried on playing. All of a sudden we started hearing the beeping of car horns, and as we looked up to the top of our street we saw that all of the cars had come to a stop in the main road, we all wondered what had happened so we ran up to take a look. There was a crowd of people in a circle in the road in front of the traffic, and they were laughing at something. I pushed through the crowd to see, and there on his knees was my dad praying in the road, in the pouring rain. I remember looking at his face with rain streaming down it, and just feeling so terribly sorry. With people still laughing and cat calling I stepped forward, walked over to him and held out my hand saying "come on dad". I remember it going quiet, my father looking in my face and saying "ok boy". I helped him up and we walked through the circle of people and slowly headed home. Without my knowing it this event had a profound effect on me. In my life I have made it my job to help any outcast person I come across, because they too are somebody's mother, father, sister, or brother, and no one will laugh at them if I can help it. This event happened during what I remember as dad's religious phase, he always believed in God but during this time his illness took control of his belief and he became a fanatical crusader for God's work, sometimes to the detriment of all else.

Shady Deals

The area where I grew up was traditionally full of what used to be called spivs, which was another name for wheeler dealers who were always out to make a fast buck or do a dodgy deal (like Flash Harry from the old St Trinians films) and I was aware of some goings on even at my young age.

A lot of the families in the area used to sell what they called dodgy stuff to each other, mainly clothing which had fallen off of the back of a lorry (in other words stolen) these goings on used to let the poorer (or greedy) people supplement their incomes, I was never aware of my mother actually having dealings with this stuff but I could not have blamed her if she had bought us some cheap clothing (as they say) on the side.

I do remember one time when it was near bomb fire night (Nov 5th), the kids in the street (including me) used to make a big event of it each year by storing up old wood for months before, and constructing a massive bomb fire on the waste ground or (bombsite) as it was still called which stood opposite my house. The whole street would gather to let off our fireworks around the fire and we would look forward to that night each year

On this particular year I had constructed a huge life like Guy Fawks dummy to be put on the bomb fire as per the tradition, and it was stored in what was later to become my Star Trek room (my sisters' old bedroom). All of a sudden we heard a commotion outside in the street and we looked out to see loads of police cars and police officers entering houses, we also heard a load of noise coming from the house next door. My mum went down to the large back Veranda which joined our two houses (which as I said before, we called the lids) to see if she could get some idea of what was going on, and as she opened the doors she saw a black plastic sack full of something outside on our veranda, as she bent to have a look at it, policemen suddenly appeared jumping across from next door. One shouted "drop the bag we've got you". My poor mum was stunned, but all of a sudden another voice shouted from another house out the back of us, "no it's ok, it had nothing to do with her, I saw someone dump it from the house you just came from".

Lucky for us the Police had been secretly watching the suspect house otherwise they would have thought the bag belonged to us. But it did give the Police enough reason to suddenly invade our house and begin searching. The only funny part to all of this was when two officers entered my sisters' old bedroom. It was all in darkness and as they walked in and turned on the light one of them became panic struck for a moment and shouted, "shit, fuck". In front of him was my seven foot tall Guy with a Frankenstein mask on and a fake axe in his hand. The police collapsed in laughter when they realised what they had been afraid of, but it still did not change our bad feelings about being invaded.

Someone next door must have panicked and tried to get rid of some stolen goods by slinging them across to our side of the lids, which was not a very nice thing to do to us. The end result of the raid was that our next door neighbour ended up serving time in prison. Our street and area was generally not a bad place to live when I was young, but as I grew older it changed.

As I was growing up the street outside my house became my whole world and because I was never allowed to venture far, it had to be. The people who lived there were part of a now by gone era, full of character and eccentricity, they also had a strong sense of community and the last time that was shown was when everyone came together for the Queens Jubilee in 1977 and then later for the wedding of Charles and Diana. As the Jubilee came closer a sense of excitement swept over the street, as I suppose it did in most streets throughout England. Every house made sure that it was fully decorated on the outside with every kind of red white and blue decoration you could think of. I painted a huge Union Jack on a bed sheet and we suspended it across the front of our house for the world to see, to be honest I plastered our top part of no 27 and it looked great.

All the parents had arranged a massive street party during the day for the children, and my mum helped to wait on tables. The atmosphere was terrific and the day ended with a stage show for the kids. I took a cine camera of the day and captured all those wonderful sights for all time. At one point on my tape my mum comes across the camera with her union jack hat on and smiles as she waits on the tables, then I pan up later in the day to reveal my dad sitting on our upstairs balcony looking over at all the happy goings on below. It really sums up his life, always on the outside looking in. On the night of the Jubilee there was a giant disco held in the underground car park of the London College of Print which was built opposite our house where the old bomb site used to be and I can remember being terrified because I had not danced since my old twisting days. I also remember sneaking a drink of Bacardi from someone out of curiosity and I hated it.

The wedding of Charles and Diana a few years later was much the same spirit in the street, only by that time I had my girlfriend Karen and we also had my niece Victoria. My new friends from Kent came up to join in the celebrations and all of us danced the night away. I remember comparing how I felt at the Jubilee to how I felt at the wedding celebrations, I was a different person. All for the better thank God. I know that that time and those days will never come again and as the saying goes, they were the best of times, they were the worst of times. Unfortunately the world and times move on, and some years later when mum went to put her rubbish out one night and opened the front door, she was pushed back into the passageway by what turned out to be an armoured and armed police officer, he told her they were doing a raid next door because an armed gang were thought to have moved in. She was kept safe and no shots were fired but when I eventually heard what happened I knew that it was no longer the street or the Elephant I grew up in.

Travesty Of Justice

My father's only recreation in his life was his piano, his occasional small bet on the horses with my Nan and his long daily walks. Every day he would dress up in his suit as if he were going out to work in some kind of office, and off he would go, usually with his little note book of secret codes to help him battle the forces of whoever, he would head for the west end of London and do his bit to right the wrongs of the World. When my dad was his sane self he really loved horse racing and once (when we could afford it) he even took me to the Derby, and a couple of times I remember going to Wimbledon and watching dog racing with him, but most of the time through lack of money his love of the sport only went as far as a few shillings bet with his mother (who still lived in 27 Oswin) when the Derby or Grand National came around. If he could not afford to place a bet his mum would do it for him (she was horse crazy).

This one year dad went to Waterloo station (which was not far from our house) to see all the people dressed in their fine Ascot clothes and hats, he always loved the spectacle and he waited for it each year. Reading this book it might sound as if Harry was strange all of the time but this was not the case, he could still interact with every day people and no one would know the fantasy world he really lived in unless he had earmarked them as one of the enemy, then you would be in no doubt that this man had a problem, and that day no doubt some people in that Ascot crowd would fall into (the enemy) category.   My dad had been gone a few hours when a knock went at our door; without looking over our balcony as she usually did, mum went down to see who it was.   When she opened the door she saw two men standing with my dad and they said, "We are police officers and we have just arrested this man for pick pocketing on Waterloo station", on hearing those words my poor mum feinted clean away (the straw that broke the camel's back).   When mum had revived the plain clothes officers said they had observed my dad acting suspiciously while moving in and out of the Ascot crowds and had seen him jostling people, they assumed he was trying to pick pocket them.   They had found no money, wallets, or purses on him but they had seen enough to warrant arresting him and coming to search our home.   As you can imagine, all of this coming on top of the life we already had was almost too much for my mum, and the rest of us for that matter.

To us it was obvious what had happened, Harry had gone amongst the crowd doing his secret signs and movements to whoever he had selected as (one on them), which to the outside world would look strange, but it was just part of my dad's paranoia and no way was he robbing anyone. During their search the police saw a plastic charity collecting tin for the RSPCA, in the shape of an old English sheepdog standing on our mantelpiece which had the bottom lid missing, they said my dad must have stolen it and used the money inside. My dad was like a magpie and used to come home with all sorts of rubbish which he called treasure, or had some significance to him. He had a drawer full of shiny beads, bits of toys coloured glass etc and he had found the dog collecting tin already open empty and discarded ages ago in St James's Park, he had brought it home for me because it looked like a lovely dog. All my life I had had it drummed into me about honesty and always doing the right thing, Harry was a man with a terrible illness but he was never a thief. There was only circumstantial evidence of his supposed crime, no stolen goods and no witnesses, but My dad was still committed for trial as a suspected thief. I know that with his imaginary world full of agents and bad guys, he may have done some strange things on the station, but certainly not stealing. All of this plunged him into a deep pit of depression and fear and he took to his bed for days at a time after that.

A London newspaper called the South London Press picked up the story and the headlines read "no job man jostles Ascot crowd". As I have said, all of this frightened the life out of my father and I can remember the night before his trial sitting on his bed talking to him, telling him that I knew he was innocent and he would not go to prison, but I was so worried inside about what the jury would think. At his trial his solicitor made no attempt to say where was the stolen money or goods, and where are the witnesses, had it been now I would have made sure he was defended properly, but in those days I was just a boy and we were as always so alone, with no money and no one to help us.

My dad's brother (Bobby) who lived downstairs and owned his own business went to testify as a character witness for him and apart from talking about my father in general terms, what he said was, "this is a sad case me Lud", that was it. The Judge said in his summing up, "I find this case reluctantly proven, you are guilty as charged". Thank God my dad was only given a suspended sentence, and because my family had no money and were so relieved he was not going to prison, we did nothing to try and fight the conviction. My poor father now had the stigma of being a thief as well as a mad man and he did not leave the house again for nearly a year, it traumatised him so much.

Two years later a Policeman who knew my mother and who also worked on Waterloo station came to see her, he had some papers with him which said that the two Police officers who arrested my dad had themselves been convicted of framing people on several accounts, also the solicitor who defended my father had been struck off for mal practice. At least the people that counted knew Harry was innocent.

Thy Rod And Thy Staff

My father very often carried an umbrella, as I said earlier (like John Steed from the Avengers) and it actually turned into his Moses like staff for a while during a period when he thought God guided his every move. One day I went over to the West End with him and this day my friend (Kevin) also came with us, as we walked along Harry suddenly hung his umbrella handle over his arm and began to stare at it as we walked, it soon became clear that wherever the handle chose to point is where my dad chose to go. We did not realise what he was up to for a while as we followed him in and out of shops for no reason, but then without warning he walked right out into the road with traffic just missing him, some swerving to do so, all because the umbrella had pointed that way, Kevin and I had the sense not to follow and he was lucky to get back on the pavement without getting killed. This seemed to snap him out of his stupidity and we began to walk normally, all Kevin and I did was exchange worried looks between us.

We were fine for a while until we came to a large window of an expensive restaurant, Harry stopped and looked in the window at all of the people eating inside, then exploded into this tirade of abuse while banging his umbrella on the window, Kevin and I did not know where to look, but that was enough, Kevin looked at me and said I'm off and with that he was gone heading back for home while leaving me with my crusading father. We then walked off with Harry in top form, pointing at people, making gestures, whistling, clapping, spinning around and saying very loudly, "you know who you are". The next stop on our traumatic journey was to what used to be the famous Playboy Bunny club on Park Lane, so my dad could again do his bit against the pornography and corruption he thought went on inside there. When we arrived the doorman eyed him watchfully as he walked up and down ranting with his trusty umbrella raised high in the air and me toddling behind him not really knowing quite what to do or where to look.

Our last stop was to the famous department store, Harrods. With my dad's suited appearance they had no hesitation letting him in (well big mistake) once we were in we went crusading from floor to floor against all of the rich and corrupt people of the world. It was a day's shopping I would never forget and never ever wish to repeat. Dad was not usually so obviously and so verbally insane in public, but at this point the curse of schizophrenia was too strong.

One day some time later he came staggering into our front room with his eye in a terrible state, mum and I rushed over to him and he told us that he had been hit by a bike in the road. He said that the handle had smashed him across the face as it went by? Well we had no reason to doubt him but we did find it a strange kind of accident to have. He stayed home for a couple of weeks while his eye got better and then he again started his daily walks over the West End of London but this time he just took a little empty note book, not his usual book full of secret signs and codes, just this blank note book. One day when he came home from his walk I saw the book lying on the table so I sneaked a look, it had nothing but timings of someone arriving and leaving somewhere followed by place names, it also had a few of my fathers unreadable codes alongside them? A few weeks went by and he came home one day looking a bit roughed up, not his usual immaculate self, but he had a strange semi smile and a kind of satisfied look, I had to ask him. He sat me down and swore me to secrecy, and then he told his tale. It turned out that weeks before he had not been hit by a bike at all, he said some bouncers outside a club did not like what he was doing (no doubt on one of his crusades) so they grabbed him and gave him a beating. I was shocked, angry and upset that someone had hurt my dad especially since I now understood that he was ill. He then just smiled and said "they will never do that again". I do not know what he did, it could have been some imaginary thing in his own mind to take care of the men who did this to him, or it could have been something far more real and physical, we will never know for sure? But maybe they learned a lesson. Beware of a man with an umbrella.

My fathers' religious phase culminated in him going missing for nearly five days. My mum was frantic with worry, she had the Police looking for him and they began to fear for the worst, but suddenly on the fifth night dad stumbled back into our front room and literally fell on top of a bowl of fruit, which he devoured like a man possessed (which I suppose he almost was). It turned out that he had walked forty miles to a town called Tonbridge (near our beloved Plaxtol) there he had blessed a school for disabled children so they might get well. Harry said he slept in fields and roadsides, and later told us he even slept in a caravan in someone's back garden for a night. He had eaten only some wild mushrooms he had picked in a field and had drank rain water collected in his umbrella. All in all he had walked an eighty mile round trip, to save children, this journey left my dad looking terrible and he was almost happy to go back yet again to the mental hospital. After all, in his mind his work was done, the world and the children were safe, for a while at least.

My Hero

Throughout all our years of trouble mum had been the one constant that never changed, never gave in and never became cynical about life. She had worked all hours as a cleaner where ever she could, she had even worked at six in the morning cleaning inside the massive local catholic cathedral school and shovelling snow from the school steps. Even though we must have been in dire straights over money, mum never let me know, for a child ignorance can be bliss.

When I was a young boy as Christmas came around I would go with mum to Woolworth's and buy packs of red, blue, pink and green crepe paper, we would also buy packs of thin wire stubs. In the weeks before Christmas my mum and dad would sit and make bunches of paper roses (I would do my best to help). My dad's family were florists years ago and used to have a shop so he knew just how to role and shape the paper into very realistic flowers. We would all sit night after night doing this, and when we had enough bunches of lovely roses the three of us would walk the streets with a pram full of our handy work, and my parents would sell them to whoever would buy. I always thought this was just one of the fun things we did at Christmas, I never realised our Christmas probably depended on it. They made sure I never knew what the paper roses really meant.

My father's real working life had come to an end with his broken ankle, and he had never signed on for sickness benefit, although due to his mental illness he would have been eligible for it long before his ankle, but you have to remember that in his mind he had never been mentally ill. So it was that the burden fell to my mother to support our whole family. After years of many kinds of cleaning jobs she managed to get a job on Waterloo station, serving tea, coffee and snacks from a trolley, the hardest part was that it was all night work, and in those days during the early seventies Waterloo was a much different place than it is today. Firstly much of the station was open to the elements and was freezing in winter, and on cold wind swept nights it was also a haven for many drunks and undesirables as well as some genuinely unfortunate people, but most of the customers were the grateful and the ungrateful public. I have said that our family was an honest one and I still hold true to that, but at one point my mum was forced to walk a thin line just to help us survive.

While mum worked on the trolley she and her co worker came up with a dangerous idea which could be seen as breaking the law, although you could argue the point. They would buy a large box of tea bags, milk and sugar and smuggle them onto their trolley at night, then at some points during their shift they would make and sell their own tea keeping the profit. They did not do this to a massive degree but in the situation we were in every little counted. I know that keeping this secret from the powers that be on the station did cause my mum a lot of strain and worry, but she did it for us. Mum's shift would begin at eight in the evening till around five in the morning, but on Fridays she would work from five in the afternoon until one thirty in the morning, so on Fridays I would wait up with my dad for her to come home and dad would welcome her with a cup of tea. I can remember missing her terribly when she would have to work all through the night, sometimes even over Christmas or New Years Eve. This went on for many years with just dad and me at home night after night, but he doted on me and always made sure I was looked after to the best of his ability, which was very well indeed. One of the things which did get me down sometimes though would be when I was watching something on TV and he would sometimes begin his conversations with whoever he thought could hear him through the box. As the years went on I learned to say, "Dad please be quiet", and he would look at me and smile giving me a nod. But I knew when I could say something and when I just had to put up with it till his mood (or mind) changed, I became an expert on all his moods and goings on and we had a unique relationship. I knew that he would have given me the world if he could and as I grew older I began to understand the tormented lovely man who lived imprisoned inside a cell of his own making, and I knew he longed for the key.

To help with the money situation but also for his own self esteem, dad would play the piano in the Prince of Wales pub at the Elephant just two streets away from our house, and people would throw money into a pot for him (he was so good at singing at his piano he should have been worth so much more) I was sensible enough to be left home alone by now but I did miss mum terribly, and remember spending many nights on my own. It was hardest on New Years Eve and times like that when mum and dad would be working and most other families would be together. I still don't really like being on my own even today, although that is how I spend much of my time, so I am kind of good at it by now.

My dad's brother Bobby and his wife Jennifer lived on the ground floor of no 27, and had done so for a number of years. Our relationship with them had been a bit strained at times when they had objected to my pram being in the downstairs passage when I was young, or to my dads piano playing. But on the whole we got on ok, they even let us use their phone to make the odd call, (which we always paid for) and also let us give their number to receive some in coming calls. Bobby had his own business and he had also been a Freemason for many years so they appeared to be quite well off. I can remember a couple of New Years Eve's when they asked me to baby sit for them (they had two boys Jeff and Martin) while mum worked on the station and dad played for the masses in the pub, and I remember how impressed I was with their fur rugs and large leather sofa, so on the odd occasion when I visited downstairs it seemed like another world to me, like some other luxury house not attached to ours. They had hot water, a shower, and their own toilet, which was a million miles away from how my family lived at the top of the house.

Because of the hours mum kept with her job she seemed to be perpetually tired, but she still did all the household jobs and looked after us, all the while still trying to keep my far from well father happy.

The inner goodness and love my mother had for everybody showed through in all she did, and I can honestly say that I have never met anyone who has come close to her with the sense of giving so much and wanting so little in return. Don't get me wrong she was no doormat and she could be as tough as old boots when the situation called for it. For Maggie Carrigan being a giving person was a choice born out of an inner strength, not inner weakness. Some of my fondest childhood memories centred around my birthdays, no matter how troubled our life was during my early years my lovely mum always made sure my birthday was a day to remember. She would save up (or borrow) enough money to have a lovely cake made for me with candles and a little cowboy or soldier on top and we would have a party with a lovely table full of goodies for all my friends to come and tuck into. I also have fond memories of my dad playing party games with me and all of my friends till it was time for them to go home full of food and fun. As I have said before, when ever they could they shielded me from just how dire our struggle sometimes was and I am grateful for that. The hardest part of her working life ended when after eleven years of braving the cold of the station an enclosed Buffet bar was built and mum was offered the job as manageress, she jumped at the chance, It was still night work but a million times better than being exposed to the elements and to danger

Although the job at waterloo was a hard one it did sometimes give my mum a chance to meet some celebrities from time to time. One story she told me was about the actress Maggie Smith who one night late for her train jumped the queue for a cup of tea, my mum saw this and asked her to get back in line, Maggie Smith then said "don't you know who I am, I am Maggie Smith" to which my Mum replied, well I am Maggie Carrigan and I am no one, so get back in the queue.

Not all of the encounters with so called famous people were bad ones though. The comedian Terry Scott often used to come up to the tea bar before he got his train home and he struck up a nice rapport with my mum. After telling me about him coming to see her I searched for a photo of him in a magazine and did a large pencil drawing for mum to give to him. When Terry saw the picture mum said his face lit up. He was appearing in pantomime at the London Palladium at the time so he gave mum two tickets for us to see the show, he also asked her to bring me round to the back door of the theatre to meet him when we arrived.

When the day came for us to see the show I was really excited because for us to go out anywhere was a rare thing, to say the least. My mum and I turned up at the stage door of the Palladium a couple of hours before the show and asked for Mr Scott, Terry was true to his word and came right out to meet us, but it did not stop there. He invited us in and took us to his dressing room where he had food and drink ready, then he gave us a grand back stage tour which ended with him placing me in the centre of the London Palladium stage. He then looked at me and said "many great people have stood here, so remember this and maybe one day you will be one of them". I never forgot that experience or Mr Scott's kindness. Sadly he has now passed away but his inspiring words stayed with me and made me want to feel that centre stage feeling again, they could have been the first inspiring words I ever heard.

The Harry Mobile

With my mothers new job as manageress of the station rail bar came a pay rise and my mum was finally able to save enough to buy Harry a car. The car they decided upon was a little Mini traveller, but if you had seen my dad's face you'd have thought it was a Rolls, this finally gave him a sense of being more like any other man, at last, his own car. The car was a part of normal life he had never had before and it became Harry's pride and joy. However my dad driving did sometimes create some very awkward and sometimes dangerous situations. Harry was a very good driver what with years of being a delivery man behind him, first for the railway then for other firms, but we had never experienced being in a car with him when the other side of Harry took over, there were many occasions when we longed for our car journey to end.

My dad would drive normally most times but if the change was upon him and someone cut him up or pissed him off in some way, Kapow. One time I can remember happening when another car cut too close to us and my dad sounded his horn, the offending driver in front did a two fingered gesture to us and that was it. Harry shifted gear and began to chase the car, and I could see he was now getting to full Harry meltdown, I tried to tell him to stop it and calm down but he was in a red mist by now. All the cars stopped at traffic lights and the target car was now a couple of cars in front, that was all it took. My dad jumped out of his Mini and hurried up to the man in the car, I could see him ranting through the guys closed window, then I saw the idiot of a driver do another sign to my dad and shout something. With that the lights changed and the cars in front began to move, Harry launched himself at the car punching the window and hanging on for dear life, he continued to punch and hang and shout as the car moved off, he was lucky that when he finally lost his grip he did not end up under the wheels of another car. The offending car driver had a lucky escape from the wrath of Harry. This was an extreme situation which thankfully ended without anyone being hurt or arrested but many trips in the car with my dad were tense eventful journeys to say the least.

Despite some nerve wracking journeys dad's little green car did become our life line and escape from Oswin Street from time to time. We had many trips to Kent together as well as days out to visit relations (the few we were still in touch with) but to dad it also meant that he could ferry me to school, or to wherever and keep me safe, which was a blessing and also a curse for me. One positive thing having the car did for me was a chance for Harry to give me driving lessons, and when he did he was always on his best behaviour, admittedly he only ever took me driving in Kent but he was still a good teacher.

The Outcast

It was the Seventies and my father had been relatively well for some time now, by well I mean he would still talk to the TV sometimes (which drove us mad if you happened to be trying to watch it at the same time) and before his daily walk over to the West End he would always write his intricate secret messages on bits of paper, elaborate codes which dad said "they" would understand. In Harry's world he fought a constant battle against the forces of evil, the bad guys, THEM, he was James Bond without MI5 behind him. But the good thing was the days of violence were gone, and the nicer Harry would show himself most of the time. He would drive a car load of us kids from the street to Kent for day trips and picnics, and on Friday nights he would drive me all over London to look at the bridges lit up like Christmas trees before we picked mum up from work at one thirty in the morning. My dad could not have shown me more love if he tried; in fact he doted on me. I grew to understand that he saw me as the perfect person, incorruptible, and one day I would be everything he could not, so I started to feel I could never let him down, or at least try not to. But the love he had for me was part of the obsession which would create my biggest problems.

Before secondary school my life had been affected by my father's illness, but not to a massive degree, I had once been diagnosed with abdominal migraine which would occasionally hit me, this the doctors attributed to the life we all had with my dad, but apart from that I was a normal little boy. As I grew older I became aware of my father's problems, and when he began to set into a dark mood I would go and sit on his lap, mum later told me that I seemed to sense that I could calm him down. But as the years passed dad's moods did start to play on my mind, some nights dad would walk around the room accusing mum of being in league with THEM and being against him, he would suddenly pull the plug from the TV and turn off all the lights, that is when mum and I would retreat off into the bedroom and sit together listening to Harry's other dark side ranting all night in the room next door. My lovely mum and I shared times like that for many years, and so we built a bond far closer than just a mother and son, we were always there for each other almost like comrades in arms, as well as mother and son.

When I went to secondary school life seemed ok, dad would take me to school in the morning then pick me up for lunch (my school was not too far from home) take me back then pick me up again when school was over, all in his little green Mini. This over protectiveness did not strike me as strange for a while, and once it actually saved me from a load of hurt. One lunch time I came out of school a bit early or dad was late, I do not know which, but as I came out of the gate I was grabbed from behind and my arm was pushed up behind my back. My attackers were three big black forth form kids from another local school who used (by tradition) to hate our school. As the three tall creeps dragged me off for a beating the little green Mini of Harry screeched to a halt and at the sight of me being dragged off, the door of the Mini flew open and fury incarnate was unleashed. Although the boys were all bigger than him, they were no match for the vengeance demon that was Harry boy in full flight. At a run and screaming, "that's my son", Harry felled the first attacker with a straight jab, the second with a fearful cross, which left the third running for his life. When my dad was losing it he always had a large Y shaped vein which protruded across his forehead, the vein was now bigger than I had ever seen it. A bystander who had seen this all happen shouted to my dad, what's wrong, don't you like blacks, she was the luckiest woman alive, as a tirade of obscenities streamed from the raging thing in front of her which was known as Harry.

When I entered the second year I moved to a new building and things started to become very hard, my dad always drummed it into me, don't smoke, don't drink, don't swear, and always do the right thing, these are all good things but they were not always the way of the real world, and they certainly were not the way of my school. My second year building had some good kids in it, but many animals as well and they all targeted me. I was very small for my age and was the only pupil to be brought home and picked up from school by his dad, also because I worked hard, didn't swear or break rules, I stood out like a sore thumb, so years of ridicule and bullying began.

At first I tried to stand up for myself, although I was small dad had taught me a bit of boxing and I remember dropping one smallish bully boy with a punch to the stomach as he grabbed me by the tie, but as time went on it all wore me down. I was kicked in the legs by a group who forced me to run the gauntlet till I could hardly walk, and a large glass beaker was thrown from an upper floor window as I walked below, exploding on my shoulder and narrowly missing my head, and that was only the beginning. It was only when mum saw some bruising on my back one day that it all came to light. She went straight up the school to the headmaster and read him the riot act, at assembly next day he made an announcement to the whole school and said, "Leave this talented boy alone". Well that was like putting petrol on a fire, the bullying got much worse and now the slaggy girls began to join in too.

Sometimes during classes before any teacher arrived one rough group of girls would flash their boobs at me and ask (in their words) "Carrigan how big is your Willy or have you got a ---- like us", all this was just to make me go red (which succeeded), then the lie went about that I was gay and I was called queer boy Carrigan. There was one girl I liked at school but even she started to join in with the taunting, so life at school became hell. All of this combined with our unpredictable home life nearly drove me to breaking point. All I had was mum, always there to tell me, "hang on boy it won't always be like this, you'll see". At one point my dad got to hear a little of what had been going on (we had kept it from him) and I came down to the playground one day ready to be picked up for lunch to find my dad pinning one of the ringleader bullies up against the wall with his nose pressed close to his face in full Harry melt down. He thought he was doing the right thing but it again only made things worse in the long run so I just stopped telling anyone about what went on at school.

One of the only good memories of my secondary school days was during my second year in 1970.

One day a man with a camera came into the playground at break time and took loads of pictures of all the kid's as we were milling around, a week or so later some of us were given a form to bring home and this included me. The form was a request for my parents to sign which would give their permission for me to be in a feature film called Melody (later changed to Swalk) the film was to star Jack Wild and Mark Lester of Oliver fame. Well at this time my dad was going through an up period, and he saw how much I wanted to do this, so he said yes and signed my form. That began three weekends of filming for me and about a hundred others from my school. It was an experience which would stay with me for the rest of my life, and from that moment on I would dream of being an actor. If only I had not come from The Elephant and Castle, and had some money and a normal father, and had... Oh well I could dream. The film was lovely and we were all invited to the premiere which was held at the Elephant and Castle Odeon Cinema on the 4th of April, which was my birthday, I went with my mum and sister and got autographs from the stars, Jack and Mark, little did I know that I would one day meet Jack Wild again under circumstances I could only dream of.

Driven To Desperation

The life I was living when dad took a particularly bad downward swing one year all became too much and at one point I was driven to desperation. Throughout this time period Harry was terrible and all our life consisted of was pain. Mum and I would listen for him to come up the stairs never knowing what he would be like, and more often than not I would see her reduced to tears as he vented all of his torment her way. I was never allowed to follow my friends to the shops or to the cinema, I was always cut off from the group as soon as they left our street because I could not go with them, my dad had forbade me to leave the street without him or mum. It may seem hard to understand now and you may ask why not just go, but to openly disobey my dad would have seemed like a betrayal to him and God knows what he would have felt or done if his golden boy had done that. So as much out of loyalty as out of fear, I just could not go against him, which meant hours of loneliness looking out of the window waiting for my friends to come back, and then feeling so out of place with them when they finally did because I could not join in talking about their adventures, all because of my father.

At that time our life just seemed one of never ending torment. Every night as we tried to watch TV Harry would constantly talk to the people he thought could hear him through all the bugs implanted in the room and in the TV, he would suddenly jump up and turn the telly off in mid programme, which was usually the point he would turn his attention to mum, that was when mum and I would retreat together to either my room or mums, to talk for hours and wait out the storm. Dad always slept on a mattress on the living room floor, so if he chose to go to bed because of a black mood, that was it, the night was over for everyone.

During one particularly long bout of Harry's mood swings which had lasted for weeks, I could see no end to what mum and I were going through. I had been in tears and said to mum, how will I ever have a normal life, get friends, girlfriends or jobs, I will be a prisoner forever. So I came to a desperate decision, although part of me loved him, I decided Harry had to die. I waited till everyone had gone out one day and I got hold of a hammer, I went up the stairs leading from my room and removed all of the carpet tacks and nails holding the stair carpet down, I wanted him to come home and fall down the stairs ending our misery, I remember waiting for him to come home down in my room in tears. Then I finally heard him, he went up the stairs and....nothing happened, but I knew the danger would be when he came down the stairs. Then I suddenly realised, what about mum, she could be the one to fall, so I rushed out of my room and quickly began to replace the carpet tacks and nails. My dad did come out to see what all of the noise was but I told him I had nearly slipped on some loose carpet so I was just making it safe. I do not know what I would have done if he had fallen, and I can't contemplate even thinking of hurting anybody now, but then again I am no longer that boy driven to desperation with no way out of a tortured existence. Thank God I held on.

The Other Side Of Harry

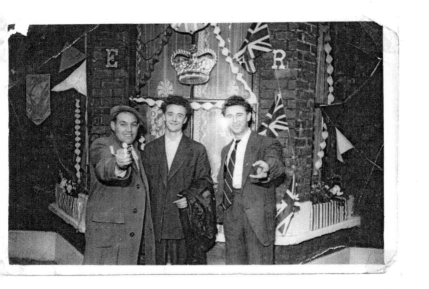

My Uncle Jim, a young Harry before the storm and dads brother Johnny at the Queens Coronation celebrations outside in Oswin Street

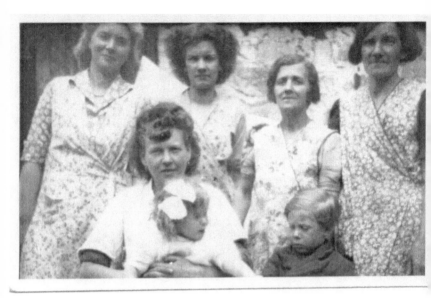

My future Aunt Iris (Uncle John's wife) mums
Sister Rose, Dads mum and Mums mum.
And in the front, Maggie Healey (my future mum)
outside the hopping huts in Kent

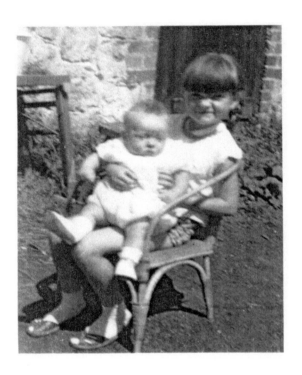

Here I am with my Sister outside the hopping huts,
my first visit to Plaxtol

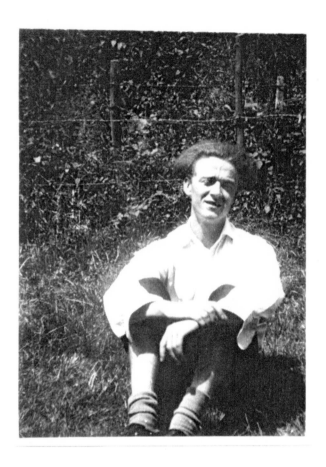

Harry in Kent after coming back to us from one of his first stays in hospital. You can see the "Y" on his forehead which seemed to appear in times of stress and acted as a warning sign of his mood swings.

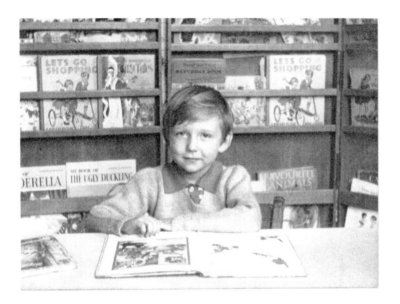

Here I am in primary school; "The Ugly Duckling"
book in the shelf behind me aptly described how I
would feel in life.

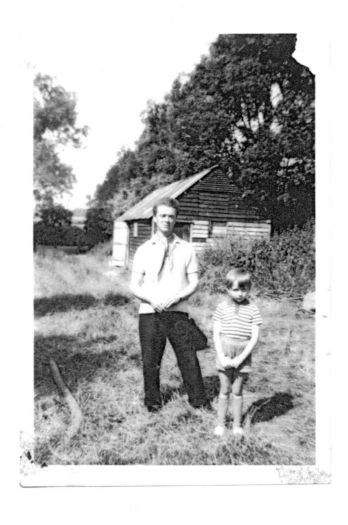

Harry and a tense little me. You can see the mood he was in and obviously so could I, even then.

The Other Side Of Harry

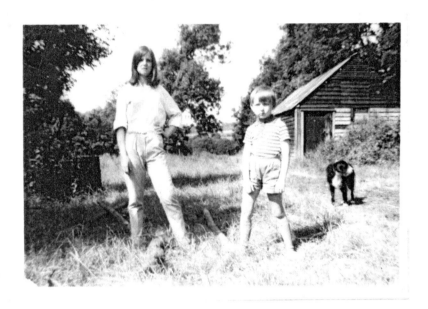

Even in those early days in Kent you could see
that Sue had beauty and poise without even
trying.
Our dog Suzy in the background.

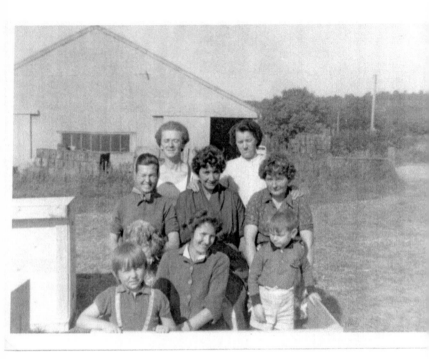

These really were the golden times for us. Here we are with our fellow fruit pickers. (We are far left)

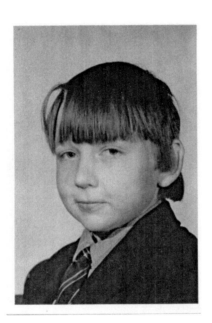

My first year at secondary school (with my home made Harry hair cut) before all the bullying began.

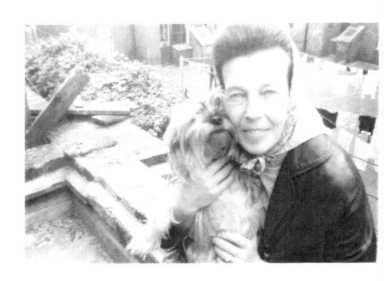

Mum with her beloved Foo Foo on our back veranda (the lids) during some really bad Harry times.

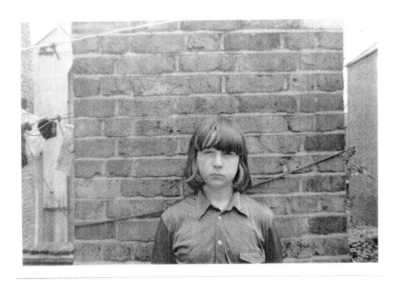

The strain is starting to show on my face as well
as mums, and I begin to comfort eat.

Leaving Me Behind

Around 1970 a new TV show aired one night replacing Dr Who on the BBC, the message of that show was that there will be a better tomorrow if we can just survive today, that message really struck a note inside me, because the thing I really needed most was hope for the future (my future). The show was called Star Trek, little did I know just what impact that TV show would eventually have on my life, I loved Star Trek from the moment I saw it, and it was to help me through many dark times through out the years, leading to something beyond my wildest dreams.

I had been with the same group of friends my whole life, Debbie the girl next door, the first girl I ever loved who only ever saw me as her best friend, Kevin my pal who shared many hours of Action Man wars with me, and later many hours discussing the fairer sex. And talking of sex, it was Kev who virtually told me everything about the birds and the bees because I never had a clue? And I knew my dad would never talk about anything like that with his perfect son.

I had started to become interested in girls, just as any young boy might do and I can remember going round to my Aunt Vi's house with my mum and finding a Playboy magazine which had been left out by my uncle Jim. After a quick glance at it I hid it under my jumper and took it home with me. I brought the magazine back the following week during our next visit without any one ever knowing it had gone. After some searching I found out where my uncle kept his stock of magazines (he owned a newspaper and grocery shop) so I repeated the process of naughty book borrowing for quite some time. Another one of my little group of friends was June. June was a sweet big breasted sexy girl who made me feel my first real sexual urges, (the first ones unrelated to my uncles' books that is). We had a grope and a kiss but were only good friends; she later grew into a really stunning looking girl. I now had my big room on the second floor of the house which used to be my sisters room, and still housed her big double bed.

My friends and I spent hours in that room playing games and jumping all over the bed wrestling (that's where my Nan got her orgy ideas). From an early age we would all call for each other after school and play out in the street till it was dark, and on weekends and school holidays we would be together none stop. Our little gang rarely left the street when we played (which was lucky for me) and our life would be one of none stop fun and games, from playing war with us boys and dying many heroic deaths at the hands of our toy guns and swords, including my pride and joy from those days (a Johnny Seven multi gun) wow, to piggy back races and games of chase with the girls. But nothing good ever lasts forever, not even childhood.

The time came when the rest of my friends stopped hanging about in the street, Debbie and June started to look all grown up and gorgeous and began to go out to pubs to look for boyfriends, and Kevin got a part time job looking after horses, picking up a girlfriend at the same time. So our days of playing action man and war together ended. I began to realise what had happened to me, my dad had never let me go out on my own, to the pictures, shopping, or anywhere for that matter, in case "they" got me. I had no idea what the real world was like and my confidence was zero. It had not helped that when I tried to protect a girl I saw being picked on in the street outside my house, the creeps picking on her then turned on me, I was head butted, kicked and nearly smashed with a paving stone, it had almost made me think dad was right, I knew he was not but I still retreated further into myself. I did not know what to do, my friends were getting lives of their own, growing up and leaving me behind.

With all I had been through while I was growing up I was bound to be affected, and although I would always try to be strong for her I can remember breaking down in tears to my mum many times, but one particular night I really was in distress as I sobbed and raged to her, "why doesn't he just die. I am fat, I will never get a girl, never get a job, he will make me a failure just like he is, I want to have a normal life". With that I exploded and punched the wall of our back bedroom and left deep knuckle marks in the plaster. It was only my mum who got me through those days by holding me and saying, "Things will get better boy, just hold on, if God don't come he sends". She had many little sayings which she would apply to life as situations arose and when I said to her, "how do you know what is going to happen in the future", she would say "God's good, you never know what's hanging till it drops". In her own way she was a little cockney philosopher.

When I look back on it now I did have some emotional problems brought on by those days, one of which was that I became bulimic. When I began to exercise and lose weight, it did get out of hand and I became paranoid about food. I would eat till I was full then go downstairs to the toilet and vomit it all up again, thankfully I did eventually stop this when mum found out, then I started eating and training my body properly. I also used to do stuff like touching things a certain number of times, which they now call obsessive compulsive disorder. These were a sure sign I had some problems because of all the stress, which thank God I eventually got control of. . But I think it was a close call and it is amazing that I am the relatively well adjusted person I am today, and even more so that I am the one people turn to for help (I think the term is a wounded healer) But I know I did and still do pay a price for those terrible days.

I began to spend more and more time in my room, I did not want to sit upstairs with my dad and listen to him talking to the telly all night so I found solace in Star Trek. I began to collect anything I could to do with the show and I eventually turned my room into a shrine to Star Trek with a massive collection of memorabilia, complete with a home made full size Captain Kirk chair and an interior mock up of a shuttlecraft with flashing control panels and views screens, my old mate Kevin spent many hours with me helping to put my mini starship together but I saw him less and less as time went by. My only social life was making Star Trek models, going through my ever growing Trek collection and drawing and painting, which I had always been good at and had loved doing ever since I was a small boy and could hold a brush or pencil.

I began to worry a lot more about my future and as always I turned to mum, but this time she could see how serious I was, no tears just calm desperation as I said, "I have no idea what I can do as a job when I leave school, I have never been out on my own further than the sweet shop around the corner, let alone trained in a job skill, I have never been out with a girl and have never even had a chance to meet one other than Debbie and June, what can I do". Mum knew that somehow I had to begin to live life so she sat down and told my dad what I was really feeling inside. In his heart the lovely sane Harry already knew how his son was feeling and also how I was beginning to look on the outside too. I had turned to food as a comfort, and the truth was, I was fat.

I had also become even more withdrawn since I was beaten up in the street (although at the time we had told Harry I had fallen off of a bike) even my dad had asked me what was wrong and why I did not play in the street as I used to. Well my mum finally poured all of my problems out to him and also voiced her concerns for my future, which must have taken a great deal of courage. To my complete surprise dad gave me the only sit down father and son talk we would ever have. He told me he would buy me some weights to help me get fit and that we would train together for boxing practice, he also said that if I was willing and good enough I could try out for art college. I cried with relief that my father had come to his senses and was talking to me like any sane father talks to his son.

He was true to his word, I sent off loads of applications to art colleges with copies of my work, and after weeks of waiting and interviews I was accepted at the London art collage Fleet Street. He also bought me the promised weights and we began to train together. This portion of my life drew to a close and I left school when I was fifteen just before the law changed the leaving age to sixteen, I had a glowing leaving report complete with seven A's and many B's, I often wonder now just what I might have achieved if I had stayed on at school, but Harry wanted me away from there as soon as possible for reasons only he knew, and to be honest, with all the bullying I had received I couldn't wait to go either.

John Carrigan

Respite From The Storm

Like Star Trek had done some years before, my life was again about to be changed by something I first saw on TV. It was 1972 and a new series came to our screens, it was called Kung Fu. As I watched the never before seen ballet like combat and heard the philosophic undertones that went with the show it fascinated me, so much so that like the rest of the country I began punching and kicking all over our house, I also started to ask deep questions about philosophy, which had to some extent also been an interest of my dad's. In many notebooks he had written down meaningful sayings such as, all of life's most important doors have to be opened with a glass key? (Think about it). Seeing value in the practices and teachings of Kung Fu (as we called all the martial arts at that time) my dad looked in the Evening Standard newspaper and found an advert for a martial arts school which had just opened in South Kensington, so he took me to watch a class, and that was it I enrolled. This was to be a life changing event.

My first days training in the martial arts school were full of nerves as you might guess, I had no self confidence whatsoever and I was far from fit, I studied a classical system called Fung Shou, I didn't choose it, it was the only class being taught at the time my father could take me. I didn't really care what system it was, as long as it was Kung Fu that was good enough for me. After I had been there for a few months I began to get more supple, and what's more it got me used to mixing with people and was so different from anything I had ever done. I loved it so much that I would come home from classes and practice all the moves I had just been taught, it was the beginning.

One night a small middle aged Chinese man sat in on the lesson and watched us all train (we had a class of about thirty at the time) and at the end of the lesson a piece of paper was given to about ten of us as we left, the paper said, you have been invited to join Master Lee Wu for further instruction in the martial arts, and a date was given for the first lesson, it was to be the first Wednesday in February 1973 and the class was called "Jun Fan Gung Fu". Good old Harry who had found the martial arts school in the first place now trusted me with these people, and he was all for me starting this new class, he even began to drop me off and came back later to pick me up, with no more sitting in on classes which used to make me even more nervous. Master Wu turned out to be a wonderful man who sought to deal with the inside of a person as well as the outside, under his guidance I took to the martial arts like a duck to water, even when I came home I would continue to train, sometimes into the early hours of the morning

My old friend Kevin came to see us one day and told both my dad and I that he had just seen a clip of someone on TV who made David Carradine on the Kung Fu show look slow, his name was Bruce Lee. My dad was curious so he did a really unusual thing; he went to the cinema all alone to check out this Bruce Lee person. When he came home he could not stop talking about what he had seen. Even though it would not be doing the right thing (as Harry had always put it) and we were too young to see the then x rated films, dad agreed we had to see this Bruce chap. So with Kevin in tow we set off for a late showing of a Bruce Lee film called The Big Boss. It was for over eighteens only but Harry sort of just hid us amongst all the crowds and we sneaked in. The film and Bruce Lee blew us all away, he was fantastic. I now wanted to train more than ever to be like him. Back in class Master Wu started to tell us more about the prowess of Lee Jun Fan, the founder of "Jun Fan Gung" Fu who he had trained with for only a short time, but that short time was enough to change Lee Wu's thoughts on the arts forever. It was only after we had been training for some time that Master Wu told us the American name Lee Jun fan had, and that name was Bruce Lee. Wow, I realised just how lucky I was to be chosen to train with someone who had actually trained with Bruce Lee. This began my quest to learn all I could about Bruce, and his teachings, including his fantastic self help philosophy. The pairing of Bruce Lee, the martial arts, and my love of Star Trek have been so important to sustaining me even today, they are and always have been my respite from the storm.

The Other Side Of Harry

My love of Star Trek also helped widen my world when one day I saw an advert in a magazine for the first ever UK Star Trek convention? It was to be held in Leicester. I still had no social life to speak of, my only real outings were to training sessions, I still saw my friends Kevin, Debbie and June from time to time either in the street or sometimes we would all get together in my Star Trek bedroom / museum to catch up on life over cups of tea, but as time moved on this happened less and less, so the Trek convention seemed to be the best thing I had heard of in a long time. My family no longer went fruit picking in our beloved Plaxtol, so it had been a few years since we had been on holiday and a chance to go away somewhere must have been as important to my mum as it was to me (the way she worked, probably more so).we persuaded my father to let us go, and even lied that we would be travelling on a special coach laid on just for the convention and Star trek fans, so we would be safe.

This would also be a monumental step for mum and I because it would be the first time we had been allowed to go away without Harry, and this would also be the first time we had seen the inside of a hotel.

When we left for our trip really early in the morning we were like excited kids on Christmas Eve, well I was still virtually a kid anyway, more so because of my up bringing, but this really meant so much to us. When we got to Leicester and into the hotel we were blown away by what people really take for granted now, our room had hot water and a bath, yippee. While I rushed all over the hotel Trekking myself silly, mum took the chance to wallow in all of that hotel luxury (a long bath). From that moment on we were hooked, and for many years to come my mum and I would go to our two Star Trek conventions per year, it was our escape and we made many new friends. In later arguments my dad would end up calling mum Mrs fucking Trekkie, which was his way of showing he did not whole heartedly approve of us going away, but he knew what it had come to mean to us so he continued to let us go.

At one of these conventions I met a man who was to help influence the direction my later life would take, his name was Rupert Evans. Rupert had been asked to the convention as a guest speaker because he had been one of England's premiere stunt men, he had the honour of having his statue in Madam Tussauds for over ten years and acted as the head stunt man for Disney Studios at the height of his career, his only Star Trek connection was that he was a close friend of Star Treks creator Gene Roddenberry.

I sat in the crowded hall and heard Mr Evans talk and saw his wonderful slide presentation of pictures and events from all of the fantastic films he had been in over the years and I found it fascinating. Rupert had had quite an amazing life even before he became a stunt man. He had been in the famous Para's during the war seeing a lot of action and had even acted as Winston Churchill's bodyguard on several occasions, after the war he had gone on to become a world famous fencing champion and had competed in the Olympics winning medals for our country. It was this fencing connection which had lead Rupert into the world of films and stunts in what has become known as the golden age of Hollywood. He was first asked to teach many of the Hollywood elite the art of sword fencing, including the legendary Errol Flynne, this then progressed to Rupert standing in for many of the stars during movie fencing scenes and at one point Rupert was even seen fencing himself as the good guy on one side of the screen and the bad guy on the other, he then went on to do all kinds of stunts in many films such as Ben Hur, Lawrence of Arabia, Treasure Island and Oliver to name a few.

I somehow plucked up the courage to talk to Mr Evans and our conversation eventually got on to my martial arts, Rupert asked to see me perform some of my stuff and he really seemed impressed by what I could do, he told me I would make a great stunt fighter one day. Rupert really did like my mum and I and took on a kind of mentoring role with me, giving advice about my training and future every time we had the good fortune to meet him, which I am glad to say was quite a few times during the coming years. Rupert was also a fantastic story teller and he would have us enthralled with his exploits about his times spent on film sets, such as when he was pushed overboard as a joke by the Beatles and was forced to swim three miles back to land while filming with them at sea, or the time he fell in love with Sophia Lorren and as he put it, made some wonderful memories. This began a friendship which would last for many years right up until Rupert's death. He was indeed a great and lovely man.

I had begun to gain some freedom and forced myself to go to shops and get on buses and trains, without asking dad's permission, but he still watched me like a hawk, and the martial arts, Star Trek and art were still all I had in my life. During one relapse the dark Harry saw some drawings I had brought home from the art college (which I attended a few days a week) and he said he saw bad stuff from "them" secretly hidden inside, just what he saw I never knew, but that was enough for him. He demanded I finish with the collage, it was not a request but a full blown raging ranting order, one you could not argue with, remember all of this stuff was so real to him. I had a secret meeting with the principle of the collage and explained the unreal situation, he said I had talent he did not want to go to waste, so we struck a compromise, I would visit the college once a week when Harry thought I was out shopping for comic books (which I loved) so I could attend a necessary class and pick up assignments to be done at home as a correspondents course. We also had any mail from the collage redirected to my Aunt Mary's house so my father would never know. I did this for a couple of years which was another strain and changed some of the course work I had to do, but at the end of it I gained my qualification in art and passed with credits, but I could never let my father know, and that was kind of sad.

It was around this time that my dad's mother fell ill. For as long as I could remember she had lived in the middle part of the house and my dad's brother Bobby lived on the ground floor with his wife Jennifer. The old lady who we just knew as Nan was also the land lady and for many years we had paid our rent to her. Well the time came when my Nan passed on (she was in her nineties) and Bobby's wife took over the rent book. Downstairs as I have said before they had their own toilet, kitchen and shower but we didn't even have hot water at the top of the house so our rent wasn't very high, it was called a controlled rent.

I do not know how it happened but the next we knew Bobby had bought the house for what we heard was a reasonably low price; suddenly we had to pay our rent to him. With my dad being the elder brother he by all rights could have been given the chance to at least buy our part of the house after all the years we had lived there. I am sure we could have borrowed the money from somewhere, maybe from one of our many rich relatives like Aunt Vi, but we were never even told the house was up for sale until dads sister-in-law

(Jennifer) came up to my mum and said that we were to pay our rent to her now. This began a problem that would one day contribute to the end of our association with 27 Oswin Street.

Life was still pretty much my mum and I and my dad's moods were still unpredictable to say the least, too many times I would be down in my room and hear dad's raised voice, forcing me to run upstairs to make sure my mum was ok, he would never touch her in those days, but he taunted her to tears many times and would be so sorry when he snapped back to his nice self. During one long bad spell when he was sure mum was getting messages via the TV and conspiring against him I had began to get really worried for mum and had almost put myself between him and her on several occasions with a new found courage the martial arts training had given me.

One day I hit on an idea which would help me safeguard mum, I installed an intercom from my room to beside dad's armchair, supposedly so I could be called up for cups of tea and stuff, but dad did not know that I could turn the intercom on from downstairs making it a one way monitor if I wanted to, that way I could listen in making sure mum was ok, and he was none the wiser. One time I even tape recorded a couple of hours of Harry upstairs alone, talking to himself or speaking to whoever he thought could hear him, just so I could get a better understanding of his deluded view of the world. I must admit that as I sat with mum listening to the tape one day, we found that we just had to laugh at some of the things we were hearing as Harry adopted a strange voice or gave an insult like, you want stuffing from you're hole to your pole, sometimes laughter was the only thing which kept the two of us sane.

Around this time a turning point of sorts arrived and I finally made a stand. My dad had begun to train with me at home which I was pleased about, it was something we could share together. Sometimes he would pick up my weights, or stretch with me and do some Yoga, this progressed on to letting me teach him some martial arts and we would hold the striking pads for each other for kicks and punches. I had only been going to the martial arts for a few years at that point but my father would watch me train and say that I could be a champion one day. As always his illness was up and down, he had it under control for the most part during the days of the late seventies-early eighties but when it gained control of him it showed no mercy.

At one such time I was down in my Trek room and I had the intercom switched on just to make sure mum was ok. I heard Harry begin to start up with his talking to the TV and then all the rest of his stuff with rantings about nothing in particular, but then he started to turn his attention to my mum. I can't remember just what it was about now but I do remember I picked up on the change in his tone so I listened more carefully. Mum tried to talk back to him and even argued for him to leave her out of it, but he then jumped into high gear. His voice became harsher and I heard him get out of his chair. That was it I rushed out of my room and up the stairs. I stood outside the living room door and listened, he was now shouting. I pushed the door open to find that Harry had his face pressed close to mums and I could see she was trying to hide her fear. I came into the room walked right over to mum and took her by the arm pulling her behind me, I then looked Harry right in the eye and said "leave her alone dad". We had a moment between us before he started pacing about across the room; he then turned to me with a face as black as thunder and said "do ya want to hit poor old Harry with ya Kung Fu, is that what you want?" I was stunned into silence but I stood firm and replied "no dad, but I wont let you touch mum, now leave her alone". He looked shocked and crest fallen, as if he had been betrayed, but it seemed to snap him out of his black mood and he went and sat back into his armchair. This marked a turning point and my dad knew from that moment on that I would always step in if he got too heated with mum, and I did. We never again had a showdown like that, and my dad never again showed the physically threatening side of Harry in our home.

High Ho High Ho

It had been several years since I left school and during that time I had only done my college work and helped out my uncle Bobby in his firm for a couple of days, on the odd occasions when he had asked me. I had also sold a couple of book covers during my stint as a freelance artist working from home, but I had never actually had a real job. This began to play on my mind because my hard working mum shouldered all our bills with her job on Waterloo Station, and later cleaning government office buildings (all night work), so I began to look for jobs in newspapers and eventually found one as a page in the Savoy Hotel in the heart of London. I can remember my first morning getting ready for work at the hotel and I was full of nerves. I had to be up at 5am to start work at 7 and for a hotel like the Savoy you had to be well groomed so I decided to use hair setting spray on my hair to keep it in place for the day. In my haste to get ready I did not look at what I was picking up and blasted my head with under arm deodorant by mistake, I did not realise what I had done until this sticky river started to run down my neck. It was too late to wash my hair so God knows what everyone thought of the pungent smelling new boy.

For reasons I can no longer remember I left the Savoy after a few weeks and moved on to working at the Intercontinental Hotel in Hyde Park, this second job involved showing guests to their rooms, paging people, taking things to peoples rooms and eventually I was also ear marked to begin training for the front reception. I had always been taught to be polite and patient by my parents, which worked well in a hotel environment, but being trustworthy backfired on me because I was then sometimes given the job of taking hundreds of pounds worth of air tickets to different hotels all over London, and sometimes I had cheques on me worth thousands of pounds. I had hardly ever been out in London on my own due to Harry, so I would be in a constant state of panic when given addresses to find by a certain time so I could deliver my valuable cargo, after a few months this proved too much for me. The years of virtual seclusion had left me so unprepared for this kind of situation. I was getting better at being out in the world but it was too much too soon. I left the hotel and felt ashamed of myself; I had let mum and myself down.

I had an uncle (Danny) and a cousin (Lynne) who worked in the print and publishing industry, so I took some of my artwork to them to see what they thought, everyone seemed to agree that I was a very good artist and my uncle promised to get me a job in the print when I was eighteen (which was not far away) well surprise surprise, that never happened As I have said I did a couple of freelance book cover jobs which gave me some money and some self esteem for a while, but they were not nearly enough to base a living on.

The Other Side Of Harry

Eventually we had good fortune smile on us at long last when the farmer who my parents had worked for fruit and hop picking for all those years contacted us. He said he owned a house in our beloved Plaxtol which had become vacant and as a thank you for all my family had done for him in the past he would like to offer it to us for a very low rental cost so my family could have a place to come back to in Kent for weekends and holidays. It was as if we had won the lottery. With mum's jobs we could just afford to do this, it had to be my mum supporting us still because my father had never claimed any kind of benefit, and since leaving school neither had I. We rented the house in Brook Lane, Plaxtol returning to the place we loved at every opportunity, weekends, holidays and day trips, and on the first day as we drew up to see our new house a song called tie a Yellow ribbon was playing on the radio, it became our returning home to Kent song and we all had tears in our eyes, especially my mum. The house also gave us the chance to return to our beloved fruit picking, which gave dad and me the chance to earn some family money, it also seemed to calm the illness which as always still dwelled inside Harry. It was a golden time for all of us.

Kent was lovely but that was only when we could get the time to go there. Life was still mum working all hours and dad up and down with his schizophrenia and for me all I had again was Star Trek and the martial arts to escape into. I still could not make the leap into a future where I could get a job, get a girl, go out to pubs or wherever, the shadow of Harry and what he had done to me as a person still loomed large. I had begun to train all hours and my body had changed from the fat little school boy into one I could be proud of, I started to buy and read many books on philosophy and psychology, I read and read so I could learn about life and the human condition, I realised that all the things I had missed out on because of the sheltered life I had lead, I would have to teach myself. They say that Buddha sat in a cave in front of a wall for ten years, and when he finally stood up again he knew all of life's mysteries (he looked inside himself for the answers) this would have to be me too. I vowed to myself that all the stumbling blocks I had encountered in my life I would turn upside down and use as stepping stones.

I had two posters on my wall at that time, one was Captain Kirk from Star Trek, sitting in his Captains chair, a fearless leader, and the other was Bruce Lee standing strong looking out to the world. I realised that without a father to look up to they had become my role models. I would look at the posters and say to people, one day I am going to push that button on Captain Kirks chair and be an instructor in Bruce Lee's school. Everyone probably thought it was just the poor son of Harry deluding himself, (boy were they wrong), my mind was made up from that moment and the past would not be an excuse for the future.

The Other Side Of Harry

A couple of years earlier my sister Sue had met and married a half Spanish chap named Gregory (Greg) and for one reason or another they now needed somewhere to live, so they moved into our house in Plaxtol. They loved it and wanted to stay, so my mum approached the farmer to ask if he would consider selling it, lucky for us he did and because of our past with him it was for a good price. Although the deed to the house was in my brother-in-law's name my mum and dad still retained some financial interest in the house, but in reality it now belonged to Sue and Greg.

Sue moved into Plaxtol with her horses (they had always been Sue's passion) and a new era began in our lives. My sister now saw a lot more of us as we visited her and Greg on many weekends and during our visits I would talk to her about my life with dad and my worries for the future. She could see what I was going through inside, I was nineteen and had never had a girlfriend and I also had no job. The only thing I was proud of was my martial arts which filled my waking hours and which I was now very good at (so I was told) but I still never had a normal life, one which Sue had to escape to find.

Without me knowing Sue asked my mum and dad to let me come and live with her and Greg in Plaxtol, it would mean a massive leap for me and a big letting go for my dad. In his heart he knew it would be for the best, it had to happen for my future, and above all else he loved me, so he said yes. When Sue finally put the proposition to me I wrestled with my conscience about finally leaving my mum behind alone with my dad. As much as she had been there for me, I had been there for her, we were a team, the best of friends and I loved her. I felt so guilty, but mum being the person she was never thinking of herself begged me to go, so I agreed, I knew I had to do it (another life changing event). I said goodbye to my old street friends, left my Star Trek collection in perfect condition for me to visit when I could and left 27 Oswin Street to start a new life, and boy did I.

Sue loved her horses and being in Kent meant that she could fulfil her dreams of owning and riding her own horses. I think that if Sue had been writing this book and chose to end on a happy note, it would be those days in Plaxtol. She also had a terrible start in life with Harry being the way he was but she got through it all to become first a beauty Queen, then a model and finally to own her own horses. So in her own way Sue had also beaten the odds to be where she was and fought her own personal battles. It took a while for me to adjust to my new life; I must admit that for the first few weeks I did kind of miss the little cocooned world I had been used to, my Trek room, my old friends, and mum. But to live free out of the control my father had forced me to live under was worth a King's ransom.

I soon got used to my new way of life and jumped at the chance to work and help out. We all used to chip in with mucking out and looking after Sue's horses, and on his visits when dad was around he also loved to join in. I can remember one time when he wished he hadn't. As he was leading one of Sues young horses (Folly) he carelessly started to let her get in front of him, all of a sudden she reared onto her front legs and kicked out with her back ones catching the unsuspecting Harry boy right between the legs, he doubled over and staggered round the garden mouthing obscenities at the horse while all we could do was stand and try not to let him see us laughing. When recovered he saw the funny side of it too, but he was lucky really, it could have been his face.

The house in Plaxtol was down a country lane surrounded by lovely fields, it was semi detached with three bedrooms and a large back garden. Our neighbours were the Burtenshaws, a family who owned a shed building firm, Burtenshaw Sheds. As part of my new life I became self employed with my brother-in-law Greg, we cleaned cars for a car salesman, did painting and decorating and went round erecting sheds and portable buildings for Burtenshaws. We worked hard and well together and things were looking up. But my new life and my ignorance of the world would soon come to cause me a big problem.

Ignorance Is Not Bliss

I really was still so naive when I began my new life in Kent, there were still so many things people take for granted that I really just knew nothing about, and this included the taxman. My working life with Greg had been going well and we got on ok, I was at last earning my place in the world, or so it felt to me anyway, I loved my life in Kent and the first year just flew by, I still saw a lot of mum and dad when they came to stay, and I would also visit them every chance I got.

As my first year being self employed came to an end a chance remark from someone started me thinking when they said, isn't it a pain in the ass preparing your accounts and books at year end? I didn't have a clue what they were talking about? I really should have asked Greg or someone who knew what they were talking about, but I didn't because I did not want to sound ignorant. So, on my next trip to London I asked my dad. Well the blind leading the blind. Because he had not worked self employed or otherwise for years he had as much idea what to do as I did (which was none) so like an idiot I went along to the tax office at the Elephant with all of my Burtenshaw, car cleaning and building wage packets from the past year or so all wrapped up in an elastic band, and plonked them on a counter in front of this woman and said, "I need to know what tax I owe, do I leave these with you?" She looked at me as if I were half witted or something and said, "er no, you need to prepare accounts", she then gave me pages of forms to fill in. So off I went back to mum and dad none the wiser.

When I got home we all sat and read through the forms, and I know it seems stupid and downright illiterate looking back on it now but dad just said, add up all you have earned and just guess what you have spent, but make sure you say a lot of it was spent on work stuff. Well I calculated my earnings and just made up a sum which I had spent, which left me with very little money to see as profit, I had kept no records and knew nothing about personal expense, business expense, subsistence, or any of the many listings which go with being self employed. Feeling I had done all I had to do I then took my form back to the tax office. A couple of weeks went by and I received a letter telling me I had to go and see the inspector of taxes, I was not really worried (ignorance is bliss, or is it?) I thought he was going to help calculate my tax…boy was I wrong.

I arrived at the foreboding looking tax offices at the Elephant and Castle and after a handshake and a forced smile the bespectacled taxman showed me to his office. "Mr Carrigan, this is the first time we have heard from you is it not?" "Er yes it is". "Are these your total earnings and expenditure over the past year?" "Yes they are". "So you spent this much on work and this much on clothes food and rent?", "yes that's right". "Do you drink or smoke?" " No I don't"…"oh really"; "Yes really, I train a lot so

I don't do things which would work against my fitness". (Then he began) "Do you buy newspapers?" "Yes". "How often?", "One a day I suppose?" "Right, one newspaper at thirty pence times three hundred and sixty five days per year comes to…" I did not know what he was doing but he went on to ask me about things I bought during the year even soft drinks when I went out, and so on and so on. When he had finished he said "where did all the money for these purchases come from, according to this you have spent more than you earn". Of course I hadn't but his questions tricked me into making it seem as if I had, I had no proof what I had spent, I had just made up a bunch of figures, he continued. "You left school several years ago but we only have records of you working for two hotels only for a number of months, how have you supported yourself". (My heart started racing and I glowed red with fear and embarrassment) "Well err …you see my dad is ill and my mum looked after us, I was not allowed out I"…(I knew how this must have sounded and I wanted the ground to open and swallow me up). He continued and literally called me a liar, saying that I had been working for years but had only now decided to pay taxes. I really had no clue! I had not lied I just had not really understood anything about being employed or self employed, since my early years I had been trapped by all that Harry inflicted on us, when I should and would have been working like the rest of my friends, I wasn't even allowed to the pictures on my own let alone going out looking for jobs, but how could anyone understand that. My mum had supported my dad and me for years and it had driven me mad with guilt, now I was at last working and paying my way I was being put through this. I finally said, "If you don't believe me talk to my mum". This must have triggered something in Mr tax inspector, he probably thought I was some kind of mummy's boy retard or something, so he said "ok bring her with you at ten o'clock tomorrow".

I went back to mum and dad shattered and explained what I had been through, dad looked like he could have stormed the tax offices and raised them to the ground, but he also looked guilty, I had listened to his advice about filling in my tax forms, and in his heart he knew it was all down to him anyway. As she always did mum said "don't worry luv, I will sort this out". The next day I had a sick feeling in my stomach as we entered the tax offices.

After we sat down the smug looking tax inspector started his next wave of attacks but before he could get in his stride the little woman beside me launched into battle, "hold it mate", she began, "before you carry on there are a few things you need to know about the life my son has led", I asked if I could leave the room while mum spoke, but the Inspector said I'd rather you stay, I gritted my teeth and my fired up mum began, it all came out, every bit of the life dad had forced me to live during the years before I finally escaped. I felt my face redden again with a mixture of guilt and embarrassment, mum finished off with, "the only thing my son is guilty of is never knowing what life should have been like for a boy of his age, he's very intelligent and talented but through no fault of his own he is also so naive about life, and as for him surviving without being able to go out and get a job, this is how we survived". With that she reached into her ever present shopping bag and slammed a pile of old school style exercise books down on his desk, each one had the words loans written large on the front, and some of them dated back years. It turned out that mum had been borrowing from money lenders all through our life just to survive, and paid back loan after loan, none of us ever knew, I was as shocked as the taxman.

He began to pick up book after book all filled with dates when money was loaned and then paid back, sometimes with massive interest, year after year. When he finally put the books down he was silent for a moment, then a change came over him as he must have realised how hard all of this had been for me and my mother. He said "I understand now, I'm sorry". It turned out he believed our story but he said he would still have to fine me three hundred pounds for past un-paid tax, he also added that if it were up to him I would pay nothing. This experience made me aware of just how ignorant I really was about everyday life, how ashamed I now felt for letting mum shoulder so much for so long, and just what a tower of strength she had been, and still was in all our lives.

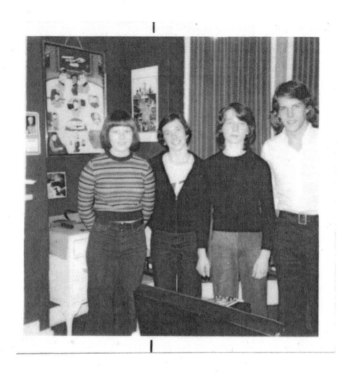

Old childhood friends, June, Debbie, me and Kevin in my Star Trek room. They were destined to leave me behind as they grew old enough to go out and seek a life and a future.

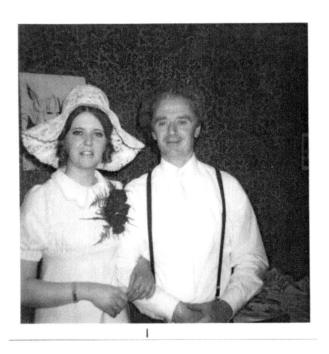

The proud Father. Sue and Harry on her wedding day

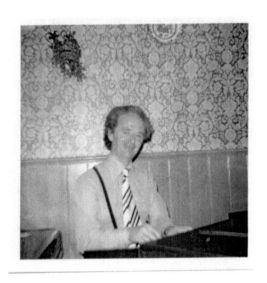

My dad happy, doing what he loved to do playing the piano

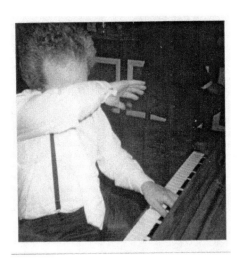

Harry sweating buckets playing for pennies in a
pub in London

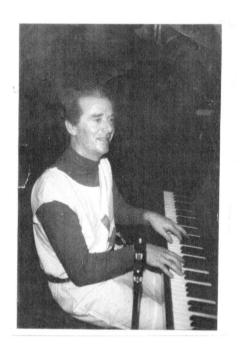

Dad dressed as a Crusader, still playing for pennies

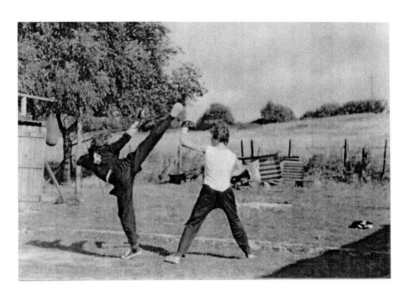

Me sparring (left) in our garden, the Shaolin
temple of Kent

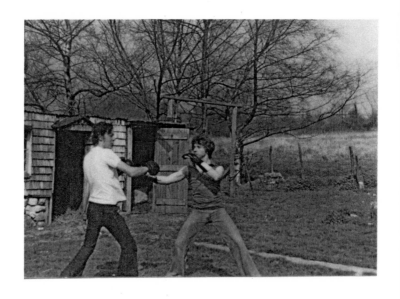

Yet more sparring and challenges (ouch) me on right.

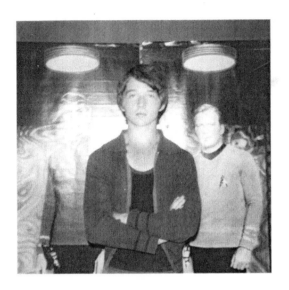

The slimline me in my Star Trek room. The diets and hours of training had paid off thank God. No more ugly duckling for me.

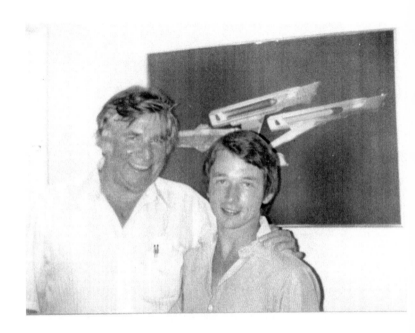

Meeting Star Trek creator Gene Roddenberry, a
life changing moment

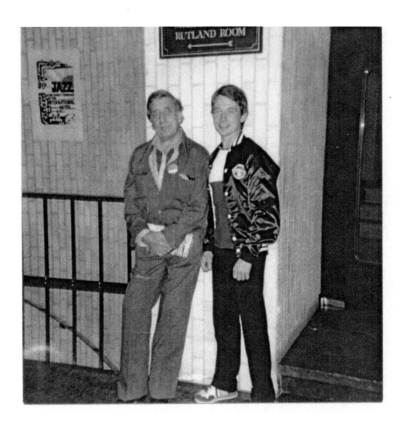

Me with stunt man, mentor and friend, Rupert
Evans

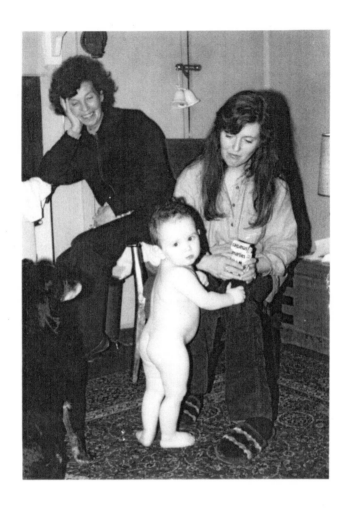

My proud mum looks on at Susan with a very young daughter Victoria, in the house in Plaxtol.

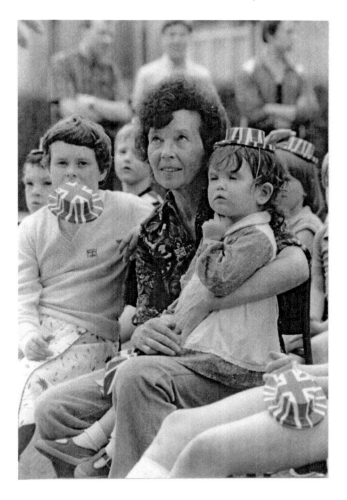

Mum with Victoria (Torrs) in Oswin Street at the
Charles and Diana wedding celebrations, with me
looking on (back far right)

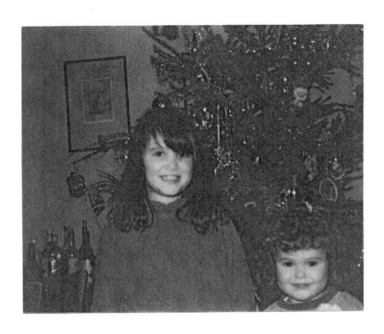

Victoria and Catalina wide eyed and happy at
Christmas time

The Other Side Of Harry

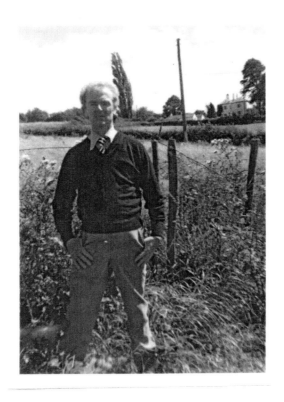

The many moods and faces of Harry, here the
dark side kicks in

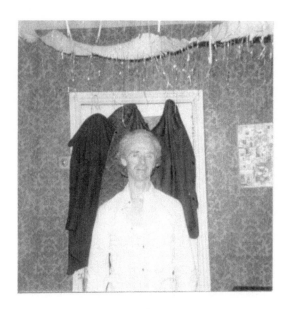

Above is the Harry we all loved, and opposite is the lonely outsider who could never find peace.

The Other Side Of Harry

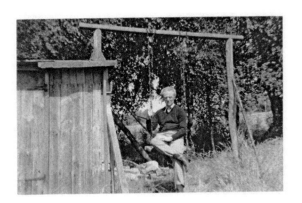

The Shaolin Temple Of Kent

After the dreaded tax fiasco I continued my life in Kent a much wiser person. As time went on I made some new friends and we began to spend a couple of nights a week doing the rounds of country pubs, (which was something totally new to me except for the Papermakers days) and it almost became a running joke that I only drank Pepsi, and sometimes my friends would order a Pepsi saying, and a Pepsi for the boy (although I was the oldest). I used to train with my weights and martial arts every night, and although I had now left the school in London I would still go back for the odd lesson or seminar and training was still a massive part of my life. I even used to travel all the way to Nottingham to train with a friend named Martin who was one of my early students. I used to give seminars at his martial arts school and would return to continue the training for a number of years.

At one time though, my training almost became an obsession. I had began training after my father had bought me some weights, (even he had to see I was fat) I also began to diet and as I have said I almost took that too far, but the fitter I became and the better I looked the more I trained. Two hours every day of the week without fail and I would only stop for a couple of days over Christmas. When times were bad with Harry training became another kind of escape and for two hours per day I could forget all my problems and focus just on myself, but as the years passed training almost took me over and by the time I moved to Kent it had to be two hours weekdays and four hours Saturdays and Sundays, this included my weights, running and martial arts. One day however after a hard session I sat down to take stock of my goals for the future and I realised I had to have a life to go with my training, so I began to fit training in with my life, not let it rule my life as I had tended to do .

People got to hear about me and my martial arts and would ask me to demonstrate. It was not long before word spread and I had people asking for lessons. The nickname Kung Fu John was started by one of my friends, a name he still calls me even today on the odd occasion our paths cross. I would give lessons in our large back garden where I had a big punch bag set up and soon it became clear that I needed to open up my first official martial arts club. This I did in a building which used to be the Red Lion pub, but part of it was now used as a pre school centre for young children, I would hold my classes after work two nights per week and I would only charge enough to pay for the rental of the hall. My confidence had grown so much along with my physical prowess that it bordered on arrogance (over compensating for the down trodden life I had lead, being beaten up and bullied) I was also so proud that I had been one of the few people (at that time) to study Bruce Lee's system, so I used to tell the world.

The word of my deeds had spread so much that people would turn up at the house from local Karate clubs and other martial arts schools, or they would just be local tough guy idiots who would all end up challenging me to fight. This happened quite a few times, mainly at weekends when mum and dad would be down for a visit. I have one particular memory of a Kung Fu instructor turning up with his entourage, and my protective father Harry boy pacing up and down the garden before the fight.

Harry knew what the martial arts meant to me so he did not try to step in, I had come too far for that and he also felt the pride I had. I was no longer just his little John I had changed inside, never again would I let myself fail or back down from life. I never lost any of the challenges and no one ever got badly hurt. I do remember one guy making Bruce Lee like noises as he came at me and acting as if he wanted me dead just before a spin kick and a punch I landed sent him crashing to his knees. As I moved in on him my mum rushed out of the house where they had all been watching, she had a tray of drinks and shouted, "here love here love have this and be friends", I think she thought I was about to kill him. My parents did not like all of this going on but it was all done in quite a controlled and honourable way, and in the end they knew I was still the good guy, I never caused the fights and they knew that I so needed to stand on my own two feet. All of this was part of me building up my own self belief and fighting my own insecurities and I desperately wanted to make my mum (and dad) proud of me.

This quest to make my parents proud was not altogether a good thing because it drove me to stupidly enter an underground almost anything goes tournament. On a trip to a martial arts seminar I had met a guy who said to me, if you really want to know how good you are you need to enter this and he handed me a flyer showing the tournament. As soon as I got back home I sent in my application and fee, the die was cast. Looking back on it now I see how wrong it was to enter the thing. In those days these tournaments were underground for a reason, people could get badly hurt or even killed, there was little regulation then, unlike the ultimate fight challenges we see on TV today (and they can be bad enough) but the insecure part still inside of me had to know, was I just lying to myself or could I really take care of myself now after all these years of training, emotionally as well as physically. I told mum and dad I had entered a tournament but they had no idea how dangerous it was. They would have done everything to stop me if they had known the truth.

I stayed in London the night before the competition and I remember the look on their faces as I left the next day, they were worried but they also wanted to let me see the faith they had in me. The tournament was held in a big hanger kind of building and was packed mostly with rough looking people who I would never have mixed with in every day life and to say I felt fear was an understatement. The life I had led and the gentle boy I had been brought up to be was not good preparation for a place like this, but my time came and my first fight was over before I really knew it. The challenger although taller than me was almost too tall for his own good, he stepped forward and threw a punch, I blocked it and swept his lead leg away, as he dropped I punched him in the face and he could not continue. The second took a bit longer because this guy was far heavier than me and got me back pedalling to avoid his heavy kicks and punches. Bruce Lee's Jeet Kune Do had taught me to use the emotions as well as the physical side of combat, so because I could see the guy was sure he had me I continued to retreat then all of a sudden I stopped and unleashed a powerful sidekick to the top of his leg as he rushed forward (we call it attack by drawing), it was over I had won them both. My opponents had been bigger than me but were nowhere near as fast. They were just crazy and ran onto the blows which put them down while consumed with wishing me dead. My last fight was against a really tall black guy in a maroon coloured satin Kung Fu uniform complete with the biggest Afro hair do I had ever seen. I had seen him fight that day and he was an animal. He had kicked a guy in the face as he was down on all fours and destroyed his face loving every minute of it, so I knew this was the one to survive. During the fight I kept him at bay using low kicks and lots of movement but half way through the fight he hit me in the ribs with a spin kick and the pain was incredible, it started to go dark and I just wanted to go down, as I started to fold I saw him coming toward me for the kill and he was laughing all over his face, I do not know what or how, but the next second I shouted "NO" and hit him with a chain of punches dropping him to the floor. I had not done it, something inside me had, and it refused to let me go down. I would never want to go through it again but I had learnt a lot about myself by doing this stupid dangerous thing.

I could only walk slowly and painfully by the time I eventually arrived back at Oswin Street but I straightened up as I walked into mum and dad's front room, I stood for a moment in silence as they looked at me in the doorway, then I lifted up my plastic golden trophy and said... I won. My father jumped up punching the arm of the chair and shouted, I knew you could do it, he rushed over and for one of the first times in my life he hugged me. I will never forget the look of pride in his eyes, my mum came over with tears running down her face and cuddled me saying, my little John, my hero. I am telling this story not to glorify myself but to show that the joy and pride mum and dad felt was not because I had kicked someone's ass, it was that for all we had been through, all we had missed out on in life, the pain, and at times the humiliation we had felt, even with all this, we could still win through. After that moment seeing their faces I knew that everything I would do, I would do for them, to somehow give them that feeling again, that feeling of pride, to let them live through me because they were a big part of me and I loved them.

Out Of Eden

Back in Plaxtol my partnership with Greg came to an end and I went to work for Burtenshaws full time, life was good. Mum and dad would visit weekends and sometimes so would my Aunt Vi and Uncle Jim (of Lambeth Walk fame) Uncle Jim was a little round man and loved his food so he would often bring loads of pies and mash and we would all pig out, the sad thing was that my Aunt Vi had suffered a terrible stroke needing surgery on her head, and she was now mentally impaired and partially paralysed, but we all still loved her and made sure she enjoyed what she could.

The house was a constant round of visitors from Sue's friends, my friends, stable girls (Sue had three horses) and our relations; it was the Walton's, almost the perfect life. I also encountered my first real feelings of love, her name was Jill, and beside an open fire with the lights low and the Carpenters playing in the background, at nearly twenty one years of age I finally found out what made the world go round. Jill and I also loved to dance together and because it was the era of the Saturday Night Fever craze we used to practice that kind of dancing quite a lot, we even won a competition dancing to the song, "More Than a Woman". Sue had loads of animals by now including, one goat, two guinea fowl, chickens, two dogs and loads of cats, so as you can guess mucking out the stables and sheds became an almost full time hobby, it was an incredible way of life. Sue had somehow also got a lovely little calf which we named Emily, she was light brown with a white chest and I swear she was almost human. Because I used to spend a lot of time with Emily she seemed to develop a fixation with me and one day I was lying on the front room floor drawing when I felt a presence, I turned around too late, to find that Emily had somehow got into the house and was proceeding to mount me from behind, I knew she loved me but that was taking it a bit too far.

I learned a lot about life during those years and I finally felt I was ready to take my place as an independent person out in the world. Mum and dad used to come down often and Greg even got my dad some work with him decorating from time to time, so the house in Plaxtol really was a saviour to us all, but as the saying goes, all good things come to an end, and so it was with Plaxtol.

My sister had a somewhat volatile relationship with Greg although they had a little girl (Victoria) and seemed to have an ideal life. One day Sue had a really swollen eye and she said the horse had caused it, I never knew at the time but sometimes Sue and Greg had violent arguments. One night a few weeks later I was reading late in my room before bed, when I heard them arguing in their bedroom next to mine, suddenly Sue called out for me in a panicked voice, I rushed to their bedroom and flung open the door to find Sue on her back on the bed with Greg holding her down with one hand while raising the other, I shouted "Greg let her go", he looked at me in a rage and shouted back, "I have had enough of you", with that he leapt up and charged at me. Greg was a heavy man and I had the stairs behind me, the next I knew he was on the floor holding his face and moaning with pain, my training had taken over and I had intercepted his attack with a punch of my own, I told him that if he carried on I would be forced to really hurt him. Well the next day Greg's eye was in pretty bad shape and the atmosphere in the house was awkward to say the least so he left for a while, he did eventually come back but things were never quite the same again. Sue and Greg's relationship carried on going down hill and Greg eventually left her for someone else and they agreed to split up.

The eventual outcome of all of this was that Sue moved to Essex where she later did have a reconciliation with Greg and they had another lovely little girl (Catalina) but after a while their troubles started again and it all ended in divorce. But the price we all paid was that our Plaxtol Shangri-La came to an end. The house was sold and mum and dad now had no place to go to find happiness, which is all they ever really wanted. I moved into a bed-sit in Tunbridge Wells with my girlfriend Karen who I had been with for some time and had just become engaged to, (my first love Jill had broken my heart some time before and moved on to pastures new). It was by no means ideal but it meant I could still work in Kent and be with

Karen. I made sure I visited London often though knowing mum and dad could no longer come and visit me, I had to make sure they knew they were never truly alone and also keep tabs on dads' state of mind. It was sad; a golden age had passed for all of us.

The Clown Prince

I continued with my working life in Kent and for the most part I loved my job and my new life. I worked for Burtenshaws at that time, mostly erecting portable sheds and buildings around Kent and Sussex. We would get orders for sheds from all over the place so we would load up the big transit van with as many as five sheds at a time to be delivered and or erected. My main workmates were the son of the boss (Steven Burtenshaw) or another long time employee (Mervyn Jons). Mervyn was a jolly faced slightly tubby fun loving mad young man, and we would have many crazy adventures together as we travelled around erecting all sorts of wooden buildings. A couple of instances of Mervyn's mad cap character spring to mind.

We had been asked to deliver and erect a shed in someone's garden while they were out, so we arrived at the address and unloaded the shed into the garden. It was a rather posh looking house with a garden to match. After we had levelled the foundation Mervyn began to put on the one man Mervyn show. It was a hot day so he only had his baggy tracksuit trousers on with a peek cap on his head. I do not know who began it but one of us started to quietly sing the 'ooby do' song from The Walt Disney Jungle Book film. Mervyn suddenly pulled his trousers up to just below his chest, turned his cap back to front and started to sing and dance at the top of his voice. Because of his shape and size, with his trousers pulled up he looked just like a Gorilla or Orang-utan. I was in fits of laughter and tears began to stream down my face as he continues to lope about all over the garden. For his grand finale Mervyn proceeded to run up a high metal pole which was part of a washing line (still full of washing). At the top of the pole he finished the song with a rousing, "I wanna be like you oo". At that moment I saw his face change, I looked across to follow his gaze and saw that large curtains had been drawn open across the large French windows to reveal the whole family from the house sitting eating lunch and staring wide eyed. They had not gone out and had seen the whole show. Well after a pause which seemed to last forever Mervyn slid down the pole and in true Mervyn style, took off his cap walked over to the window and held it out for donations. With that the tension vanished and the whole family exploded in laughter and applause.

Another Mervyn stunt unwillingly got me roped in. We were again erecting a large shed in a lovely stately looking house which this time was owned by two lovely old ladies. As I brought the first shed panels around to the back garden I saw that they were at home and were having tea behind their French windows, as I passed by I nodded and smiled and they smiled back. I started to level the base for the shed and I heard this tapping, I looked up to see Mervyn walking past their window with a thin cane out in front of him, he was staring blankly in front while tapping the floor as he went. I saw the two old ladies look at each other as he went by. By the time he got to me they had opened the window and were coming over to us. Mervyn had bent down and had the spirit level in his hand, he was feeling it while looking up to the sky, again with this blank expression. "Oh my dear one of them said are you alright"? Mervyn turned looking past them and said "yes I am fine thank you. I am the only blind shed erector in Kent". They looked at me and said "this is amazing, how does he know when the ground is level enough for the shed?" I was committed now, "It is a special brail spirit level" I replied. "Oh how wonderful" they said back. Well the rest of our job that day saw the lovely old ladies bringing us cups of tea and cake, while Mervyn continued to awe them as the blind shed erector. I felt so guilty when they came to see us off at the end of the job; they gave us a five pound tip to share. But the rotter Mervyn had not finished. He jumped up into the driving seat of the transit van still staring with un-focussed eyes and prepared to drive us away. One of the old ladies looked in awe and said "how does he manage to drive"? For a moment I was lost for words till Mervyn reached out of the window with his piece of Cane and started tapping the floor. I looked at the lovely old lady and with my best actor straight face I said, "We're a team". He started up the van and I began to say, "Left a bit Merve, right a bit, carry on forward". As we drove away I saw the two old ladies still in awe waving to us as we went. That was Mervyn. My old workmate has since passed away, but he still makes me smile and will never be forgotten.

Normal

Part of this book is about how a life like the one we had with my father is bound to leave scars, and for want of a better word demons, but not all demons have negative effects.

While living in the bed-sit with Karen we would talk about our future married life together while struggling to pay our bills. Karen and I had a passionate but volatile relationship with many arguments. We would come home from work, have our meal together and I would go off into the hallway of the building to train (the only place with enough space to move). I had always said to people around me, "I can't stop my training; one day I will need it I know I will". I did not mean just to defend myself, something in me was calling me and telling me, these hours, months and years of training are for a reason, don't stop. During one of our arguments I just came out with – "I can't sit watching Coronation Street or just go down the pub after work, this is not who I am, I don't want a so called normal life, I am going to be different". I had said it (I was different), I did not smoke, drink or follow football, I was into philosophy and martial arts, I still loved Star Trek. I had my own views about never being a follower, and being who I am.

I dreaded being "Mr nine to five", I had a morbid dislike for that kind of life, for me it seemed like the kiss of death. I felt I had to and would prove to myself and the world that I would make something wonderful of my life, and take my family (mum dad and Sue) along with me, a drive which had been forming within me for some years now. That drive is why I had tested myself with all my training, teaching, the tournament, and travelling around the country, I had to prove myself to myself every chance I got, but that became one of my demons. At times it has made me push too far, but more often than not it has pushed me to succeed. It can be a heavy burden, always wanting and needing to succeed at anything I do to the point of seeing any kind of failure as a stigma, and as I grow older I find that feeling still within.

Dexies

It may be hard for anyone who did not really know him to see my dad as anything more than a nasty man, his illness could and often did turn him into one, but a lot of the time he was a lovely person and we did spend many happy times together.

One good memory occurred during the time I was living with Karen. My Uncle Jim bought another shop just around the corner from Oswin Street and wanted to renovate it, Harry had been well for some time now so my uncle asked him if he would like to earn some money and do the job, I knew the work would be too much for one person and my dad needed the money, so being self employed in Kent I took the time off to help my father. I moved back home for two weeks and we began, we had to gut the whole shop, rebuild new shelving and paint and make good everything, we also had to knock out an old bathroom which was part of the house attached to the shop. We really worked hard together and although it was a dirty rough job at times we did spend loads of quality time talking as father and son while we worked. Karen also came to stay during the weekends and joined us in the shop. The flat above the shop had a lovely piano in and I can remember one day hearing my dad playing it and Karen singing along with all her heart as the two of them did a duet.

When we finally finished the shop it looked great and soon after a pop group called Dexies Midnight

Runners brought out a hit record called "Come on Eileen", and they filmed the pop Video outside the shop and it was seen all through the Video. So our work was immortalised for all time. Those two weeks were lovely memories of how things might have been if Harry had not been cursed with his illness, and it showed that we would have made a great team as father and son. But one thing was to sour all the work we did. Because we had done such a good job my Uncle Jim offered dad a job serving in the shop and also picking up goods from the cash and carry. On top of that he also offered dad a maroon hatch back car, and said that if dad insured it and had it put through a mot, he could have it. Harry was really pleased to be trusted with a job and over the Moon to be offered the car. Mum paid for it to be insured and put through a mot and dad went to work in the shop, he also began making runs to pick up the goods and would return with the car full to the brim. After a few weeks my uncle got another man in to manage the shop and asked if he could borrow the car. Dad was never asked back in the shop and he never saw the car again. This time the failure was through no fault of his own. He was just, as they say, sold down the river.

To Boldly Go

Once again being the only break she would have my mum and I continued to go to our beloved Star Trek conventions together, which gave her a chance to relax and meet up with friends she had made at the conventions over the years. Mum was not a Star Trek fan as such but she liked it and the people who were at the conventions were our kind of people, mostly searching for some kind of escape from a hum drum or troubled life and looking for a better tomorrow, so we fitted right in.

A few years earlier there had been a problem at one of the Conventions when a large crowd of football fans went on a rampage right outside the convention hotel almost trampling a disabled girl from the convention, I managed to get her inside the hotel using some of my martial arts skills and held the doors closed to prevent crazed football hooligans wreaking havoc inside the con until Police arrived. As a thank you for my actions I was allowed to go to breakfast with the con guest, George Takei (Mr Sulu) I also went for a run with George and struck up a friendship with him. From that event I was then asked to be low key security at many Star Trek conventions, and I ended up looking after all of the original Star Trek cast members at one time or another, including my hero Captain James T Kirk (William Shatner). One lunchtime I even got to exchange some martial arts moves with him.

I had been doing this at conventions for a couple years when someone named Richard Arnold came over as a guest. He was the assistant to Gene Roddenberry the creator of Star Trek. During the con I got to meet Richard and we got on very well, we continued to keep in touch when he returned to LA. I continued my life of putting up portable buildings for Burtenshaws, living with Karen, and trying to make sure mum and dad were ok, and all the while I continued training and training, but inside I still felt I had not yet found who or what I was going to be.

On one weekend visit to see mum and dad my aunt and uncle downstairs received a phone call and it was for me (they still let the odd call come through for mum and dad) Jennifer called up for us and I went to take the call. It was Richard Arnold calling directly from Paramount Pictures in Hollywood. Richard said that he had been speaking to Gene Roddenberry about me and he had told Gene all I had done to help the Star Trek cast members at conventions over the years. Gene had asked Richard to call and invite me over to Paramount to meet him and have a tour of the Star Trek sets. Can you imagine, coming from the Elephant and Castle with the life I had led, loving Star Trek the way I did, and having an invitation like this. At one time leaving my street seemed an impossible dream, let alone leaving the country for Hollywood and Star Trek, add to that finally not having to worry about what Harry would say, it was like a miracle. I told Richard I would love to come over (as if I would ever turn that chance down). I had to get myself a passport and a loan for the air fare but thankfully Richard had offered to put me up during my trip which would save me a load of money. Mum and dad were nervous but very happy for me, so I was set for the trip of my life.

Hurray For Hollywood

I was excited beyond belief about my trip but also apprehensive, up to a couple of years prior to that I had never been on a bus on my own let alone a plane, and because of my fathers irrational control over me I had only ventured a couple of streets from my home, now I was about to go thousands of miles. Thank God I had started to break away when I did otherwise I could never have managed to take on a trip like this.

My first flight was fantastic, and nearly twelve hours after take off I landed in Los Angeles, Richard was there to meet me at the Airport (phew) and off we drove through the city to his home, past palm trees and the shimmering sights of Hollywood. During my incredible first trip Richard made sure that this boy from the Elephant saw all the wonders of California, including Hollywood, Las Vegas and the Grand Canyon, but the main focus of my trip was to go to Paramount and meet Gene Roddenberry.

On the day we drove along Melrose Avenue and through the archway of Paramount studio's gates I felt as if I were in a dream, we parked the car and headed for the Star Trek offices. When we got out of the lift and walked into the office the first person I met was Susan Sackett, Gene's other assistant, but almost before I had a chance to say hello to her there he was, Gene Roddenberry. He was a very big man, well over six feet tall with a shock of shaggy silver hair and a smile as wide as he was tall. Richard introduced us and I reached out to shake his hand (typically English), Gene bent down and gave me a massive hug of welcome, I was speechless, he then said, "come into my private office and lets have a chat", with that we left Richard and Susan in the outer office and went to have the chat which would change my entire life (my second life changing event).

Follow Your Dreams

I sat in front of Gene's large desk and marvelled at all the Hollywood trimmings around me, including all the Star Trek bits and pieces around the office. Gene poured us both some wine (I was not going to say I don't drink – I drank that day) and after talking about my life and his for quite some time we arrived at that life changing moment, Gene looked me in the eyes and with a smile said, "what are your ambitions John", I thought for a moment and said (like some Trekkie idiot) "I would love to sit in Captain Kirks chair", he grinned and said, "well we can do that for you, but what are your life ambitions", I smiled and without any hesitation said, "I wish I had been an actor", his face became serious and he replied, "are you dead?". I was puzzled and said with a smile, "no?" Gene then said "well why aren't you an actor?" I stated what I thought was the obvious answer and replied, "I can't act". Gene leaned forward and looked me straight in the eyes as he said, "if man had only dreamed of going to the Moon but had not taken the steps and the risks, and strived to get there, we would be Earthbound, if you wish to fly tomorrow you must flap your wings today". "When I was a small boy I used to put cardboard boxes on my head and pretend they were my spaceship, when I grew up I called that spaceship Enterprise." He then put his hand on my shoulder and said "if you really want to be an actor, follow your dreams and take the steps you need to take, a better tomorrow begins today".

He smiled a lovely smile at me and I did not know what to say. Then he said "let's fulfil that other ambition."

I was then taken to the Star Trek soundstages by Richard who gave me a fantastic tour of the Starship Enterprise. When we entered the heavy soundstage door the studio was in darkness and Richard led me to a spot and told me to stand still with my eyes closed, after a few moments he shouted, "open your eyes," as I did two doors in front of me slid open and I was staring wide eyed into the corridors of the Enterprise herself, all lit up and looking one hundred percent realistic, he then said "now come on board" as I stepped forward the doors closed behind me and I was inside a place I had dreamed about ever since I was a young boy. As I carried on walking along the corridors Richard would shout , "now turn right," as I did another door would slide open as I got to it and I would imagine the swishing sound I had heard so many times on TV, (Richard was up on the catwalk controlling all the doors as I got to them). I walked through engineering, sickbay, and the transporter room, (where I just had to stand on the platform and beam down, wouldn't you?). Finally I stepped out of the elevator and on to the bridge. There in front of me was the Captains chair, I walked up to it and remembered what I used to say to people about one day pushing the button on that chair, I looked at the arm full of buttons, had a moment to myself, then I finally pushed that button (done, ambition number one) before promptly sitting myself down in the Captains chair. Pushing that button had shown me that the impossible is possible (sometimes).

Before I left the studio Gene gave me a special certificate signed by him which he usually gave to VIPs, including NASA Astronauts stating that I was officially a member of the USS Enterprise crew, it is something I will always treasure. Later in the trip I went to dinner at a Chinese restaurant with Gene and Richard, it was plain to see that this was my first time eating Chinese food so Gene Showed me how to use chopsticks, and even fed me with a smile now and again till I got the hang of it, He was a truly lovely man, and a great talent in the world.

Although my main reason for going to the states was to see Gene and the Star Trek sets I could not let this chance pass by. Bruce Lee had lived in Los Angeles and opened up a school there, after his passing in 1973 some of his students had got together to carry on Bruce's teachings and keep his name alive (as if that were ever needed) so I took the chance to visit the IMB academy which was run by sifu (teacher) Richard Bustillo, one of Bruce Lee's friends and original students.

I met sifu Bustillo and after talking to me he must have seen something which sparked his trust and friendship because he then gave me a grand tour of the academy which ended with him showing me some of Bruce's original training equipment.

Before I left Richard offered to take me on as one of his students which I gratefully accepted (I had officially become a second generation Bruce Lee student) which I considered a rare privilege.

My instructor Richard would visit England many times in the years which followed, not only to train me but to teach at seminars I had organised, and I would also go back to LA many times to continue my Jeet Kune Do training. Since my first meeting with sifu Bustillo I have trained with many of Bruce's friends and students and eventually after over 30 years in the martial arts I earned a full instructorship in the IMB academy, which would fulfil my second ambition of being an instructor in Bruce Lee's school. I still have the two posters which began my ambitious dreaming all those years ago and they still act as a reminder to me that faith backed by action can move mountains.

The Star Trek Bruce Lee journey continued.

A Goal In Life

I came home from my first trip to Los Angeles a changed person, and I would never, could never be the same again. I now had within me a burning ambition which had its first stirrings many years ago when I filmed Melody, this ambition had now been fanned to massive heights by Gene's talk with me, I would be an actor – no matter what, How to go about it was a different story. I was still living with Karen but we had problems, the fire which fuelled our love also sought to consume it. The problems between us grew till we both knew our getting married would never happen, we had gone as far as booking the date of the wedding but that is as far as we had got. Karen got fed up with waiting and found someone else (who she eventually married) we had been together for nearly eight years so as the song goes, breaking up is hard to do, and it hurt.

I moved into the house of one of my long time friends (Ron) who I was also working for at the time doing all kinds of back breaking work, from building to demolition to tree felling to cesspit digging, we did them all. I later moved to share a bed sit with another friend of mine (Robin) who made Casanova look like a Trappist monk. It was fun in the bed-sit, but at times it could be a nightmare.

Once when I came home from work Robin had some friends round for a drink and they were a strange looking group to say the least, but I was the last one to judge a book by its cover. I sat and let them get on together happy to be a bystander just making small talk, until one of them started to unroll some silver foil, he then got out this stuff which looked like a large lump of brown hard wax. As I looked on he then got out a lighter and the group gathered around him. That was enough for me, it was not my flat but I could not just stand by. I jumped to my feet and said "What the hell do you think you are doing, no one is going to take drugs in front of me in a place I have to live in. If the police crashed in here right now we would all get busted including me".

They all looked at me stunned, then one of them who was on crutches said "I am disabled man and this is all I have got in life to help me through". He then continued to get ready to (as they say) 'Chase the Dragon'. I pushed my way into the group and grabbed the lump of stuff. I went over to the back window and threw the lump out into the garden. I turned on the group of five and said, tough, but not in front of me. Robin was not into drugs but he looked as stunned as the rest. I think he must have told them about my abilities because all they did was just mumble to themselves before leaving into the night to retrieve their lost crap. Robin had not followed them, he stood just stood looking at me. I said I was sorry to do that to his friends but there are some things in life you must take a stand on, and for me that was one of them. He just smiled and said "shall we have a cup of tea?"

My flat mate was quite a character, he had built a bed on scaffolding right up next to the ceiling and his antics reminded me of how a spider would take his prey high up into his web (Robins prey were women) which he frequently did while I shared the sofa with Robins dog down below. That dog and I spent many sleepless nights fighting for space on our luxurious bed. Other lovely nights were taken up trying to dry my soaking wet work clothes by the little electric fire ready to put back on next day, and sometimes they would still be damp by the time I had to get ready for work. I was no saint during those times and I did see a couple of girls while living at Robins, but nothing compared to the steady influx of girls who shared Robins scaffold bed night after night. I had to be up at five in the morning and sometimes I was still awake at three am listening to the screams of joy drifting down from the lofty heights of Robin's love nest, these were hard times in more ways than one.

Star Ceremony

I lived in Robin's bed-sit for more than a year and one of the two good things to happen during that time was my meeting a lovely girl called Lynne at yet another Star Trek convention and she was to play a big part in my life. Since my break up with Karen I had gone off of the rails a little (as you might put it) and used my new found confidence to charm quite a few girls, you could call it making up for lost time, I was no Robin but I did some things I now regret, but meeting Lynne changed all of that.

Lynne lived in her own flat in Reading and at that time was awaiting a divorce, she was a lovely strawberry blond with beautiful flaming hair, she was like a breath of spring coming into my life, and could you believe it, she loved Star Trek. The other good thing which happened to me during that time was when I received a Gold embossed envelope from the desk of Gene Roddenberry himself inviting me to be a guest at the Hollywood Walk of Fame where Gene was to receive a star on the sidewalk (pavement), with the invitation was a letter from Richard Arnold saying that my expenses for the trip would be paid for as Gene's guest, and that I should not feel guilty about it because I would be working as part of the security for Gene and all of the Star Trek cast who would be attending. I felt so honoured and again could hardly believe it.

On my first trip to meet Gene I had spent quite a bit of time with him, including lunch at the studio and dinner at the Chinese Restaurant, but being invited to his big day in Hollywood was incredible. To cover all the things I did on that second trip would be impossible, but let's just say that Richard and Gene made me feel like a star as I first helped get the Paramount studio sound stage ready for the party, drove to Hollywood Boulevard in a stretch limo to stand with the rest of the Star Trek cast and VIP guests, then went back to Paramount for the party, WOW. After the fantastic party I took a moment to walk up to Gene and thank him for all he had done for me, as I turned to leave he said where are you going, now I want you to come to my other party in Bel Air. With that I was whizzed off to my second grand Hollywood party, only this one was especially for Gene's friends, I was doubly honoured.

At the party it was almost too much to take in, what with the champagne, the caviar and all of the people from the film and TV world that loved and respected Gene. I recognised many faces from show business (as well as the Star Trek cast of course) such as Peter Graves the white haired lead actor from the original Mission Impossible series; he had been a friend of Genes for many years. One particularly lovely moment came when Nichell Nichols (Uhura from Star Trek) sat on Genes lap and sang a song specially written for him, called Gene (funnily enough). It was an incredible night. During these trips to visit Mr

Roddenberry I got to know several of the original cast of Star Trek and over the years I would spend many happy hours at breakfast, lunch or dinner with them and also be privileged to see them work while visiting the set of many of the Star Trek movies. Every time I went back to England after one of these trips, back to my normal life (as normal as life could be for me) it became clearer what I had to do, I somehow had to break into the world of acting.

The Voyage Home

Trying to fit back in to normal work and life became harder and harder, I was still living with Robin and seeing my lovely Lynne whenever I could, which meant frequent trips to Reading or London for stays with mum and dad, (who loved Lynne), but the hardest part of all was the job I was still doing with Ron, all back breaking manual work. One day all the stress of being in a job I hated came to a head when during an argument with Ron on a building site I lost my temper and threatened him (all six foot three inches of him), he was my friend but also my boss, so it was not the wisest thing to do. Ron sacked me right away but in doing so he also gave me a talking to I have never forgot. He said that I annoyed him because out of all of our circle of friends I was the only one who had the chance to really make something of myself, I had all of these talents such as being an artist, a Kung Fu expert, and I had studied all this philosophy stuff, and now I even had friends in Hollywood, but I played it safe, and would only work for people like Ron for the rest of my life, and that's what pissed him off.

All of this had the ring of truth and had been in the back of my mind and heart for years, that had been part of the reason I had exploded at Ron that day, I was angry with myself. Now hearing it from him so soon after hearing Gene Roddenberry tell me to follow my dreams was the final straw, the catalyst I needed to spur me to action. I packed my bags and moved back to London with mum and dad, but this time it would be to find a way to begin the life I had dreamed of, not go back to the life I had left when I first moved from Oswin Street.

In the few years since I had last lived at home with my parents I had changed so much in so many ways, hopefully for the better. I was much more confident, had a lovely girlfriend and now also had some experience of life out in the real world. It did feel strange to be back in my old Star Trek bedroom but in a way it also felt good, because now I had a purpose and a goal in life and could contribute to mum and dad's lives to pay back for the years they had looked after me. I had always felt guilty about leaving mum alone with dad, knowing how he could be during his bouts of illness, now I could at least be company for her again and give her a shoulder to lean on for a change (not that she ever would). I knew that in many ways it had been hard for them since I left and inside mum and dad were pleased to have their prodigal son back. The first thing I had to do was find a job, any job just to get enough money to pay my way, not a career job, just one for now.

There was a hotel just across from the end of our street called The London Park Hotel and I saw in a local paper that they needed a laundry person, (not a glamorous job I know but remember I had dug sess pit's before now) the advantage was there would be no travelling to work involved, I could nip home for lunch and be back in work five minutes later. After a short interview I got the job which consisted of going round the many floors of the hotel with a large trolley and picking up all the dirty towels and bundles of sheets left outside the rooms by the maids, we then had to throw all the bundles down shoots which led to the basement of the hotel so that we could then sort and bag them up to be sent off to be cleaned. I worked with two other lads much younger than myself, one (Chris) had just left school and the other (Martin) had been there for a few years, everyone knew and liked Martin because he was a really lovely soft spoken Irish chap who would not say boo to a goose, and even though it sounded like a cliché he really did say 'top of the morning to ya'. It soon became known that I was someone a bit different when I hung a large sack full of discarded towels up in the basement to use as a punch bag during breaks. I also went to the hotel manager and asked for gloves and dust masks for myself and the boys. The dust and particles from the sheets and towels filled the basement as they crashed from the shoots above and all kinds of muck (and I do mean muck) was plastered over the sheets and towels, so who wanted that on their hands or in their lungs, I could not believe someone had not asked for some kind of protection sooner.

As word spread in the hotel about the little martial arts laundry guy people started to ask for lessons, and I obliged for a bit of extra income, I also did a couple of commissioned drawings which also drew in some cash. I continued to go to see Lynne or she would come to see me which was the only thing which made the hotel bearable, but I had not forgotten just why I had come back home in the first place. Each week I would buy a newspaper called The Stage and TV today which was aimed at people in the entertainment industry, I also began to seek out the places where actors got together to see what contacts I could make.

The time came around for yet another Star Trek convention with my mum, I still went with her because she loved the social side of the cons so much and they were the only break she ever got, but now I took her, not the other way around, and the difference was we were no longer alone, Lynne completed our convention trio. At this con one of the guests was a young British actor named John Shackly from a series called Tri Pods, during the con I got talking to him and the martial arts and philosophy came up, John was a Buddhist and he said he wanted to study the martial arts, we hit it off right away and a friendship grew. I began to teach John the arts and he also invited me to a Buddhist meeting. The form of Buddhism John practiced was not all about putting on robes and shaving your head, it was a modern form of the practice which aimed at getting rid of all forms of negative feelings from within you, and was meant to spur you on to positive action.

A Positive Attitude

Going to the Buddhist meeting with John felt a bit strange at first, because as part of their meeting they used to sit and chant together, I later understood that they did not chant to a deity or God but to something they called the mystic lore of life, this chant was really a rousing cry against all the negativity we carry around inside of us, and was a way to create a positive attitude followed by positive actions. I met many people from the entertainment industry at these meetings (which is one vocation you need a positive attitude in), although I embraced the positive attitude and chanted from time to time, I was brought up as a Christian and had a strong belief in God (although I did not go to church). So, I still to this day consider myself a Christian Buddhist (I believe in God, and myself). Because many people in the Buddhist circle were from the industry and included some really big names they got together to put on a musical production at one of the big London theatres, and they wanted to include a martial arts style dance routine. I did what was to be my first audition and got the job of choreographing that segment of the show. Once I had been in the theatre and felt the tingle of performance I knew with all my heart I had found where I wanted to be.

A Test Of Belief

I had been back in London for some time now and all during that time I had looked for a way to get into the industry, but I knew you needed an Equity card to really get anywhere in those days. To really get a chance of getting a card had been made into a catch twenty two situation, you needed a card before you could work in the film and TV industry but you needed to show some work before you could apply for a card? One day I was passing a magazine rack in a shop when I saw a martial arts magazine, on the front cover it said 'do you want to be a martial arts stuntman?' wow this is just what I had been looking for.

My days with Rupert Evans, my old stuntman friend, came flashing back to me with all the things he had taught and told me. One of the first things Rupert had ever said to me was "you will make a great stunt fighter one day", I had to buy it. I read the article which showed a stunt team who were going to hold a stunt course and show all the tricks of the trade, this course was to include a weekend test before you could be said to have passed and one person would be chosen to become part of the team with a view to earning a coveted Equity card. This all sounded fantastic but also daunting and I almost did not pick up the phone to book onto the course, but with all of the positive attitude I had worked hard to acquire I summoned up the positive vibes and before I knew it I had booked the course. I knew part of the test was to include screen combat including martial arts, so I knew I had to be in with a chance on that score, but the rest of it was an unknown entity, all I knew for sure was that I had to be in the best shape of my life.

The course was two months away so I began to step up my training and one lunch time I was sprinting from home back to the hotel where I worked and I came to a small fence between the road and the hotel. As I always did I leapt over the fence in mid run, but as I landed on the grass I heard a crack and the world seemed to explode. I was falling and as I rolled over and came to a stop I looked down to see the sole of my foot starring up at me completely turned over. I instinctively grabbed my foot, pulled and twisted it back into place while still shouting in shock and pain. As I had landed my foot had gone down into a small hole which had dislocated my ankle badly (the same thing my father had done years before), the pain was incredible and I literally had to drag myself the rest of the way to the hotel.

When I eventually got help and was taken to the hospital with my ankle the size of a barrage Balloon they found I had badly dislocated it and had virtually snapped all the tendons at the same time. I was put into plaster and given crutches, I could not walk so I could not work and for the first (and only) time in my life I had to sign on the dole and collect unemployment benefit. I could not believe what had happened, my dreams of getting into the film world all hinged on my doing well on the stunt course now less than eight weeks away and I could not even walk. I fell into a deep depression and even though mum and dad tried to cheer me up I felt as if (for the moment anyway) all my dreams had been shattered and I would be in dead end jobs for the rest of my life. On hearing about my bad news I had a visit from my actor friend John Shackly, and I vented how I felt onto him saying, "a fat lot of good all the chanting for positive energy has done me, look I am virtually a cripple", John replied, "this is fantastic, the best thing which could have happened to you". If I could have reached him I might have knocked him out, (I ranted) "how can you say that, being my friend you know just what that stunt course means to me, what it could have meant to my future, now that chance has gone". John calmed me down and proceeded to tell me that in his Buddhist teachings they say, any good venture full of positive energy will be challenged by the negative energy of the universe, it is the yin yang principle of opposites, he then said that one energy can be used to create the other and these challenges can be a good thing. I said "oh great and that is supposed to make me feel better", I was in with a chance of winning a place on the stunt team before my accident and now it was impossible.

The word impossible seemed to spark a memory in John so he began to tell me this fable; 'The arrow and the rock'. One day back in history a father was working out in the fields while looking after his young son and it began to get very hot, so he sat his son behind a large boulder in the shade while he carried on working. As he continued his work he moved some distance from his son but every now and then he would look over in the direction of the rock and hear his son playing behind it, but on one occasion when he looked up his heart missed a beat as he saw that above the rock was a large wolf perched on a ledge waiting to pounce on his son, the father was too far away to reach his son in time so he grabbed his bow and arrow from his back and quickly drew back on the bow string, but it was too late the wolf leapt from the ledge out of view down behind the boulder and onto where his son was, the man let out a terrible desperate cry and fired the arrow at the rock. The arrow went straight through the rock and into the wolf killing it and saving his son.

All the people from his village got to hear about this fantastic feat of firing the arrow through the rock which seemed (impossible) so they asked him to show them and do it again. The proud father once more drew back his bow and let fly – the arrow bounced off of the rock, he tried again and the arrow bounced off again. I was confused and said to John, "what does that have to do with my situation?" John replied, "The man could only fire through the rock because "he had to" to save his son, the terrible situation had made him achieve the seemingly impossible", he then went on "now your foot is the terrible situation and the stunt course is the rock, can you imagine how you will feel about life if you can still pass the course and make the stunt team even with this disability? After that nothing in life would seem impossible, but you will have to pull back your own bowstring like never before to go through that rock (because you have to)".

I have never forgotten John's words or that attitude to life, because it had always been my mum's attitude with which she had survived almost impossible odds to get us through life, although she had never explained it in a fable. As the weeks drew on and my ankle slowly began to heal I continued to sign on for unemployment benefit and hated it, I received a couple of letters from the hotel asking when I might be ready to come back to work, and would I be able to continue doing all the heavy lifting the job involved. In their own way they were beginning to apply pressure.

Throughout all of this my girlfriend Lynne had been very supportive. Travelling down to London every chance she got, sometimes on a week night after work which meant she had to go back at the crack of dawn next day. My mum and dad thought she was wonderful and so did I, she understood all about my dad and just let all of his eccentricities wash over her as if they never existed, which with the way Harry sometimes was had to be no easy task. She fitted right in with all of our sometimes strange goings on, and I could not wait for her divorce to come through so she could really be mine.

My Arrow And The Rock

The time came for the weekend away at the stunt course in Manchester, I had undergone a lot of physio at the hospital and now only had a slight limp, I had even began some light martial arts training, I was not my old self but I was ok. One of the main problems (apart from the pain) was the fear that my ankle would go again in the middle of a kick or jump which I knew would have to come on the course and that would have been the end. Doctors told me that I had just missed having to have my foot pinned so I could not afford to do it again. But this was it the time had come, so with my foot heavily bandaged and full of pain killers I went to face the arrow and the rock.

When I arrived at the hotel in Manchester I met the head of the stunt team Brian Sterling, he was well built, sun tanned with blond hair and dark glasses and his girlfriend looked just the same, they seemed to exude what every one thought a stunt person or an actor should look like. The rest of the team had the same larger than life kind of attitude but they were all nice friendly people. The other attendees on the course varied from martial artists who were champion this or champion that to people fresh out of the army, and a couple of other 'wannabees' who had never really thought it out and never trained in any way but just thought they could be a stuntman.

The first day of the course consisted of demonstrations and classes with the experts on acting, firearms, high falls, fencing, fire stunts, and finally screen combat. We all worked really hard and some of the opposition was really good, some others should never have gotten out of bed in the morning, especially one girl called Judy who instead of relaxing and flopping over onto her back during a high fall, froze on the edge of the building for ages before finally jumping, and when she eventually did she went stiff as a board and plummeted face down, nose diving through the mass of cardboard boxes leaving only her feet visible sticking out at the end of her dive, she was ok except for a bloody nose. I thought I had done ok during all of the tests so far because I put everything I had into them and ignored the voice inside me which said, don't jump off of this high thing or don't let them set you on fire, I just went for it all the way (the arrow) but by the end of the second day my foot was killing me. We were told as a finale we had to put together a scene using as many of our skills as possible including screen combat, and we would be using other members of the team as our cast.

As I thought about what to do I saw many of the others using this as their chance to show the world they could be the next Bruce Lee and during rehearsals they were kicking, punching, jumping and throwing them selves all over the place, and some were very good at it, I knew that with my foot the way it was I could not compete on their level. Then something Bruce Lee had said came to me, he said "the mistake people make is to see a person and then go and try and imitate them, you should always remember to just be yourself". So I put together an act which included plenty of action and combat but also comedy, it was a comedy martial arts spoof, although it contained some of the best martial arts my foot would let me do, including some nunchaku's (clubs joined with chains) I also included a great deal of me being me and making fun of myself, which gave everyone a good laugh, it also gave me a chance to show that I could act. By the end of the course I was limping quite a bit but I had survived and fired my arrow as hard as I could at that impossible rock, all I could do now was wait to hear the results. When I arrived home mum and dad were pleased to see that I was in one piece and to be honest so was I. That night I can remember sitting with my foot up resting and looking over at dad in his armchair with mum sitting on the floor between his feet, he was softly scratching her head for her as she drifted off to sleep. It was something she had always loved him to do.

Dad had been a lot better over the last couple of years and it had given mum the chance to again get closer to the man she fell in love with. She still worked so hard every morning cleaning government offices at Saint Catherine's House, which was the offices of births, death and marriages but she was no longer out all night (mum had left Waterloo after sixteen years of night work), but with mum being mum she had also become a carer and looked after two elderly women who were sisters (Bell and Emma) and sometimes when they went on holiday or in hospital we had to look after their foul mouthed minor bird (Deno) who drove us all mad. As I sat looking at my parents I wanted more than anything to help them and to give them something to be proud of, they could not do it so it was up to me. A couple of weeks went by and I received a letter from the hotel saying that considering my lengthy absence and the uncertainty of my being able to do the required job on my return they were going to have to fill my vacancy, so in short I was being fired. It was a shock in a way but also a release.

As fate would have it a couple of days later my Aunt called up from downstairs saying I had a phone call. I went to answer and found it was Mr Brian Sterling the head of the stunt team. Brian said I had impressed all the team members and if I wanted it he would like to offer me a job as part of The Stunt Action Service show team, to begin working with them early in the New Year. I was over the moon and of course said yes. I ran up the stairs and just exploded the news to mum and dad, their faces lit up and mum cried, I then put on the record FAME and we all did silly fame type dancing all around the living room, Harry had us it tears of laughter as he did impressions of Max Wall and Mick Jagger as he danced, at last we had something to celebrate. My dad laughing and dancing was the side of Harry we all loved and had missed for so many years. During this time we did see more and more of the lovely man inside him and it was never more evident than when my sisters two little girls (Victoria and Catalina) came to visit grandma and grandpa, there would be screams of laughter as Harry would chase them with the end of his umbrella calling himself Mr Hooker, they loved him.

Riding the crest of this great news I took the moment to propose to my girlfriend Lynne who had just received her final divorce papers, and lo and behold she said yes, maybe our lives were beginning to look brighter at last.

A Home Of My Own

Lynne and I sat down and seriously talked about our future, we both agreed it was time to try and get a place together, Lynne lived in her own flat and had a good job in Reading but we had spent many happy times visiting old friends of mine in Kent and they had in turn become her friends too, she knew I loved Kent and had heard all of the old Plaxtol stories, she had also spent a couple of New Years Eve's in the Papermakers pub with me so she was no stranger to all my old haunts. We both agreed that this part of the country was the place to begin our new life together if we could.

We started our house hunting and Lynne put her flat up for sale, I had lived in Tunbridge Wells for some time and knew it well, so that was where we went with our estate agent fever. As luck would have it we saw a small two bedroom house in a part of Tunbridge Wells called Toad Rock and we fell in love with it, with the money from Lynne's flat for a deposit it was right in our price range, we had to have it. All the documents were signed and a date was set for us to move in, we could hardly wait. I knew I would need a flexible job so I could still pursue my dreams of being in the industry and I even thought about working for Ron or Burtenshaws again, but that would have felt like a step backward, and I still remembered Ron's talk to me about working for people like him for the rest of my life just to play it safe. Then it came to me, the one thing I had spent many years training in and sacrificing for, the one thing I even had trophies to prove I was the best at was, the martial arts. In Kent a lot of my friends already called me Kung Fu John and at that time the martial arts was still a massive part of my life, Lynne had faith in me and had moved her whole life to be with me on that faith alone, so I would have faith in myself as I had taught everyone else to do, I would teach the martial arts for a living and open my own school.

By the time we were ready to move into our new home It was well into a new year and we were both so full of excitement and hope for our new home together and I felt a special pride because I was about to live in the first real home of my own. But fate moves in mysterious ways. We were within a couple of weeks of moving when I received a phone call from the head of the stunt team, it was time to go and join them in Manchester to prepare for the tour. I was filled with so many mixed feelings, this was the start of my dream but I would have to leave Lynne behind, I would not even be there the day we were to move into our new home, it seemed a big price to pay. But cometh the hour cometh the man. Harry stepped up to the plate to save the day, it was my dad's chance to help us and to feel needed, he didn't let us down. While I headed for Manchester racked with guilt and sadness about leaving the girl I loved and missing out on what should have been the first wonderful nights in our new home, Harry was the hero. He drove a hired van to Reading and with a couple of my friends moved

Lynne all the way to Kent, then he stayed over night to help her unpack and safely settle into her (our) new home. My dad was great, the father he always could have been if only his illness would have let him.

There's No People Like

My plans for opening a martial arts club would have to be put on hold because my first contract with the stunt team was for three months, which seemed a long time but when I arrived in Manchester I began to feel at home very quickly. The members of the team were great, there were only about a dozen of us in all but the team certainly had a close knit family kind of feeling. The first tour I was to do was in conjunction with the Co Op Bank. We were to tour the north of England in an open top double decker bus visiting a different town almost every day, we were part of the bank promotion which included putting on live stage and stunt shows, acting as security for celebrities hired for appearances by the bank and also jumping into a large cute bear suit as Berty the Co-op bank stunt bear, (I seemed to be the best Berty so I usually got the job).

Sometimes the team would be part of a large Carnival procession which included the team bus led by Berty the all dancing high kicking Bear (guess who) and on blazing hot summer days the heat inside the costume was almost unbearable (pardon the pun) this was all to get people to open accounts with the bank on the spot, usually accompanied by some free gift or another. Among the many different tours I did with the team was a trip to the Highland Games in Scotland to put on a stunt show at the Worlds Strongest Man event in front of thousands of people. It was great to meet these strong guys in person and to get to spend some time with them. It was a gruelling event with our team putting on martial arts demonstrations, as well as fire and car stunts. The jobs while on the team were many and varied, and one job we all looked forward to doing was when different model agencies would ask us to run self defence courses for the girls on their books, which would mean at some point in the course having to lie on top of some gorgeous girl to show her how to escape such a situation (hell of a job but someone had to do it). We would also sometimes help people to make world record attempts for the Guinness Book of Records and one of our team actually broke the world one arm push up record by doing thousands in one hour.

You never knew what job you may be called upon to do next so you really had to learn to think on your feet and stay ever ready. With the team base being in Manchester it gave me the opportunity to go to the actors centre housed in the Granada TV studios, those drama classes became the first of many actors centres I would visit around the country to improve my acting skills. The great thing about the work we did was that some of it could be put forward when the time came to gain the much sought after Equity card, after all we were acting in front of thousands of people during our tours and I really felt that I was slowly becoming what you might call a true performer (others might call it a ham). Being away from Lynne and my family and friends was almost like being suddenly drafted into the army and I had to be totally self reliant and focused on what I was doing (a far cry from the lost boy I once was staring out of my Star Trek room window).

During the times I spent away I grew enormously as a person but looking back on it now I must say that not all my changes were for the best. Inside me a feeling had begun to grow, I loved the life on the road and being in front of the crowds far too much. After my first three months tour I came home to Lynne and Toad Rock (I had only been able to rush home for the odd weekend during the tour) I was back living in Kent in a home of my own and with a lovely lady to boot. I was lucky that Lynne was the kind of person she was, I had left her to move into our new home all alone, in a place where she had no real friends (they were all mine) and she had not complained once, but deep inside I sensed that she had begun to resent the industry for taking me away from her, and she had a right to feel that way, it was a sign of things to come.

Lynne had landed a job in the accounts department of a food company in Tunbridge Wells and she seemed happy, I found a large hall I could rent for a couple of nights a week to begin building my martial arts classes and after putting the word out for a couple of weeks I organised an opening demonstration night. When the time came for the demo, (as always) the crowd who turned up were a mixture of people, some had just come to see what this little bloke had to offer and some (the so called hard men) had just come to try and make a fool out of me, or as the saying goes try and put one on me. But I was secure in all my years of training and by the end of the evening I had a hall full of believers and a good list of people for the first classes (which included some hard men with bruised ego's). In a short time my club grew and I began to feel secure in the fact that I could earn a living this way (until stardom arrived at least) and I also felt that our new house had grown into our home.

As soon as we could we invited my mum and dad down for a visit, it made me so happy and proud that I could at last bring them back to their beloved Kent, and into my own home, we also visited my sister and nieces who were living in Essex and brought the girls back to stay with us for a visit. On one trip to my sisters we came back with a lovely little smoky grey and white kitten who we named Merlin (because we thought he was a magic cat) he became our pride and joy. Later we also gained a lovely little black kitten that ran right up the curtains the moment she arrived so we called her Ninjy, naming her after a Ninja.

Life was good and continued with us both working hard to build our home and also make sure we kept an eye on our parents, (Lynne only had her mother now, her father had died just after we had met). I continued to go away on tour with the Stunt team every few months and then had to come back down to Earth to resume my other life, which was proving harder and harder to do. We still went to our Star Trek conventions and once a year flew across to visit our friends in Los Angeles. On one trip I met a woman named Paula Crist, she was a stunt woman who had worked on Star Trek and another sci-fi series called V, I struck up a friendship with her and helped arrange for her to come to England to be a guest at a British Trek convention. Paula wanted to put on a stunt show at the con so I put together some of my friends from the martial arts and some from the stunt team to do the show with us, the stunt show was such a hit that at the next convention I was invited back as a guest in my own right, and that was to be the beginning of my being a guest at many conventions over the years (which I still do to this day). Eventually I put together my own stunt show team called "Heroes for Hire" and we did many great shows and conventions, we also raised a lot of money for charity at the same time.

One funny happening at a convention involved my mum. I was a guest at a con in Shepperton where the guest list included, Dave Prowse (Darth Vader from Star Wars) and George Gibb (a double academy award winning special effects expert) and none other than, me. I had choreographed a stunt fight scene to do on stage as part of my presentation, and I had taken along "big Steve" (as we called him) Steve was part of my "Heroes for Hire" stunt team and he was to be my large opponent for the fight. Mum as always had come to the convention with me and I had sat her in the front row to watch my show, it was going to be great.

Steve and I kicked, punched, fell and rolled across the stage before moving on to swords. Steve was supposed to disarm me and my sword would land behind me, I would then backward role, pick it up and win the day. As the big climax approached and my sword flew backward landing behind me, I began to walk back at the point of Steve's blade. Just as I was about to role I heard …"Look out son, don't step back, there's a sword behind you, you might fall over it". I tried to continue but… "Watch it boy it's behind you son". I looked down to see my little concerned mum waving at me to get my attention. At that point I just had to do it, I shouted "stop" to Steve and held my hand up. I turned to the audience and said, "Has anybody seen the film called 'Stop or My mum Will Shoot?'" (A lot of people raised their hands) Then I looked down pointed at mum and said. "Well there she sits". The crowd exploded into laughter. (The film starred Sylvester Stallone and he was about a police man whose mother used to keep showing up while he was on patrol to look after him). Then I turned and looked at mum saying "I know the swords there mum, I put it there mum, I am not going to fall over it". The audience thought it was hilarious and carried on rocking with laughter. I then said "now stand up and take a bow." This she did to great applause, and then I said, "I love you but now sit down and be quiet." Again the laughter echoed, I shook my head and carried on with the fight.

A couple of years went by and we had made our new house into a home, I had begun to make a living from teaching the martial arts and I had also spent several months out of each year on the road with the stunt team doing live theatre, promotions and stunt shows. I now had enough contracts under my belt to be put forward for my Equity card so I crossed my fingers and sent off my application. After what seemed long weeks of agonised waiting I at last heard back. I had been granted an Equity card (YIPEEE). I had put in quite a few years training now as both an actor and a stunt performer and at last I felt ready to try for a career on the screen, but I knew I would have to start at the bottom to both learn about the industry and earn the success I so longed for.

I had become very close to my stunt team boss (Brian) over the years and he had heard all of my stories of visits to Gene and the Star Trek sets, so we decided that we would both go to LA and I would introduce him to all my Hollywood friends, and who knows what great contacts he might make.

I contacted Richard Arnold and we arranged to stay with him during our trip, which would save us a load of money. It turned out to be a great turn of luck for Brian because by chance a casting director who worked on Star trek The Next

Generation spotted him in the street and thought he would be great for an episode filming the next week, they needed blond body builders (which Brian was) to be used as aliens. I was really happy for Brian but inside also a little sad that I could not be involved. Gene Roddenberry himself drove Brian and me over to the costume department so Brian could be fitted for his costume. While I sat there beside Gene watching the fitting he suddenly called over the head of costuming then told me to stand up and turn around. Gene then said "what do you think? John looks like Starfleet material to me". I stood dumbfounded as the costumer said "I think so too". I was then fitted for my own Starfleet uniform. I could not believe it; I was going to be in Star Trek too.

But to cut a long story short, sadly I was eventually ordered off of the set during filming because unlike Brian I had not been put through by the union, I was only there because I was a friend of Gene's. I had to fly home to leave Brian filming, which really upset me. But I had actually made it into a Star Trek uniform because Gene Roddenberry himself thought I was good enough. So close yet so far.

When I came home I went on one more tour of shows before sadly bidding farewell to the Manchester stunt team and set about the next stage of my dream. I had bought the Stage and TV newspaper for some years and I knew they often listed agents who were seeking people to represent, I knew from talking to actors that getting an agent was no easy task they could be very choosy, but I thought I had to at least try and get one. I knew I needed to get some experience of being in front of a camera, which was totally different from being on stage, so I would apply to join an extras agency. I had some professional photographs done and found an address in the stage paper to send them off to. The agency I had found was called Elliott's and they were based in Brighton, now all I could do was wait and hope (the story of my life). A week went by and I received a call to go for an interview, at last it had begun; now the rest was up to me.

By the voice I had heard during that first call, I was expecting some large Hattie Jacques kind of woman, but when I actually met the lady from the phone call she was totally the opposite. Her name was Marcelle Elliott, the head of the agency, she was a small grey haired lady with glasses who perpetually chain smoked, but what a character she was, although it sounds like a cliché, Marcelle did actually call everyone darling and was so much larger than life. As it turned out she loved me and signed me up right away.

Throughout the years I was with Elliott's Marcelle was very good to me, and career wise I owe her much, sadly she is no longer with us but like many people from the show business world her memory lives on. The first walk on job I did for Elliott's was a small bit on the (then new) TV series called The Bill, I just had to walk into shot among a group of people and shake my head when asked a question and I remember when it came on television I sat watching as if I had a leading role. I phoned up all of my friends to see if they had seen me and glowed with pride when they said they had. I taped my first screen appearance (of course) and took it up to London to show my mum and dad, they had seen me already but we still replayed it a couple of dozen times just to make sure, I just wanted to see their faces and although a part of it was ego and I loved the thought of being on TV, at the heart of it was the fact that I would always be doing all this for my parents first, and myself second, making them proud was what counted to me.

A Jobbing Actor

Over the next couple of years I did loads of extra and walk on parts, the difference being that an extra is really a moving piece of furniture, a face in a crowd so to speak, where a walk on is when you are a lot more featured, sometimes on your own and you can even be given a couple of lines to say. Marcelle had two kinds of people on her agency books, the people who were just there to make some money and only ever wanted to be an extra, and then there were people like me who could act and dearly wanted to become an actor.

One day Marcelle phoned me and said that she was putting me into what she called her A list book, and from now on I would only be put up for good walk on spots or small parts, she also knew of my stunt back ground and before long a few parts came along where I was called upon to do some simple stunts such as doubling lead actors in a few BBC series, I also began to get jobs with quite a few lines here and there.

An embarrassing and at the same time lovely story which springs to mind was while filming on the series "The Darling Buds of May". I have mentioned the series before in this book and at the time it was very popular on TV, one of the reasons for its popularity was a beautiful young actress named Catherine Zeta Jones (who is now very big in Hollywood and married to Michael Douglas). I had a fan boy crush on her as did most other red blooded young males and I wondered if I would get a chance to see her on the shoot. I was playing the guy who ran the lift up to the cliff top in some coastal resort like Hastings and I only had one line. I was on the beach front and thought I had a couple of hours before I was due to film but a production assistant came running over to me and said that my scene had been brought forward so I had to get ready now. There was no time to get to the changing rooms so I was told to get changed on the big old unit bus (the place where we all had our dinner) so I grabbed my costume and jumped on.

The bus was empty and had curtains so no one could see me getting changed. I stripped off to my underpants and peered out between the curtains as I got ready wondering if Miss Jones was anywhere to be seen (I just wanted one glimpse of her). All of a sudden the hair on the back of my neck stood up and I felt that I was not alone. I slowly turned around to see Catherine Zeta Jones standing on the bus smiling at me as I stood there in my bright green underpants (yuck). She said "I am terribly sorry, I wanted to go to the toilet and I was told that this bus would take me back to the hotel, I did not know you were on here" (I felt my face turn burning red) I replied "no problem I will jump off". I struggled to get my trousers back on and put two legs in one almost falling over. Catherine came down the bus and put her hand on my shoulder to steady me (I wanted the ground to open up). As I fumbled to get my trousers on and not die of embarrassment she gave me a kiss on the cheek and said "you are a true gent". I jumped off of the bus and cringed off down the beach. I had got my wish and then some, but for her to see me like that, OH MY GOD.

The biggest job I had in those early days was on the children's classic series of The Chronicles of Narnia which involved going away on location to Derbyshire and Wales for weeks on end, and I loved it. One of the stars of Narnia was an ex Dr Who (Tom Baker), I got to know Tom quite well and shared many nights visiting the local pubs in the heart of the Derbyshire countryside. The other leads on Narnia were children and one of them was a rather precocious little blond boy named David, he used to be very friendly with everyone but could also be a pain in the ass. My character was a Narnian rock man guard and I had to wear an all over rubber body suit with armour on top of that, and sometimes we were deep down in underground caves in very cramped claustrophobic conditions, and being encased in rubber and armour could sometimes be a real test of nerves and stamina. Young David would delight in taking our swords from us and insisting that he wanted to fight the Narnia guards. One day when I was not in my costume David saw me kicking and punching around on my own, that was it, Kung Fu Kung Fu Kung Fu, he was my little friend for life.

When Narnia finished both Lynne and I were invited to visit David's home and meet his family, I also arranged for him and his whole family to visit Paramount studios in LA when they went out there for a holiday. I became David's martial arts instructor and he would come and visit us for training in Tunbridge Wells, I kept in contact with David and he trained on and off with me for many years. David has grown into a young man now and we still keep in touch, he lives and works in LA for a major film studio and is doing very well.

My early TV and film career was very much a learning time for me, all the walk on and extra work helped me to watch and learn many tricks of the trade. By sitting and taking notes of all that was going on around me I learned all about the camera set ups for, close ups, master shots and cut aways. As well as that I also learned about hitting your marks and minimalising your actions on camera which would prove to be invaluable to me over the coming years. I also watched many great actors up close and learnt the art of acting for film as opposed to stage acting, which I had chosen as the main focus for my career. My drama classes had been great for the craft of acting, but learning just what the camera needs from you is a very 'hands on' experience. I did all kinds of TV, from game shows to sitcoms to dramas. I even did some live Christmas specials which were always great fun. I was also fortunate enough to have a small part in a film with the famous old comedian Norman Wisdom, the film called Double X was to be his first none comedy role and it was a dark gangster movie. I played a gang member who was lined up against the wall and shot, which brought into play my stunt training (and lots of fake blood).

Life continued with me teaching in my school and taking small parts on TV and film when they came up, but I began to feel a change taking place inside me, I felt restless if I had long periods without any film work and I would bring that feeling home with me to Lynne. I was now teaching my classes in the middle of a lovely remote farm surrounded by green fields. I had rented then renovated a large old barn type building turning it into a great martial arts club and training ground, the only problem was that it only had one cold water tap, no toilet and no heating. I would teach private lessons all day and then hold my club class at night, it was lovely in the summer but freezing in the winter, and sometimes after eight hours of lessons I would feel utterly drained, soaking wet with sweat and longing for home...and the film industry. Although I loved the martial arts I was beginning to resent teaching it day in and day out. One day scanning the industry magazines as I always did I saw an open audition for a martial arts film due to be shot in Birmingham (of all places). This was the chance I had been waiting for, for years. I went off to Birmingham full of nerves but also full of determination.

The producer of the film was a chap named Bey Logan, I had heard about Bey for years, first as a martial arts magazine editor and then a martial arts agent and film producer. Bey tested all the applicants and filmed us going through our various fight scenes, at the end of the audition he announced his choices of people for the cast, and lo and behold my name was among those called. This was to begin a long association / friendship between Bey and myself which led me to work with him on Hong Kong style martial arts films and become part of the Beymark Hong Kong stunt team. Over the years I had become a person who just could not stand back and be part of the crowd, I was not pushy but I was eager to show what I could do and on many TV shows films and auditions I would seem to do well and make some kind of lasting impression which often led to friendships, this happened with Bey. He came to stay at my home in Tunbridge Wells on several occasions and we worked on a number of projects together, he is now a big name in the Hong Kong film industry and when he visits the UK we still as they say, 'do lunch'.

If I could have seen into the future when I was younger and someone had told me that I would one day live in a lovely little house in Kent, with a loving girl, have my own martial arts school and work on bit parts in films and TV I would have thought that all my dreams had come true. But I had changed a lot since being that lost boy in the Elephant and Castle retreating into my Star Trek room to avoid the troubled world brought on by the other side of Harry, and I was still changing.

My lovely Lynne seemed happy with her job, her house, her cats and me, she once told me that she did not need a hobby, I was her hobby, she had all she needed, except marriage. We had been engaged for a few years now and to Lynne it was time we were married. I had felt these changes coming over me since my stunt team days, they were an exciting time in my life, touring from place to place with people who felt just the same as I did, and there were girls, lots of beautiful girls, dancers, models, and actresses. I had not cheated on Lynne but I had been flirting like mad and had felt myself being tempted many times. When I had come home from touring I felt I had less and less in common with Lynne as the industry played a bigger and bigger part in my life.

I remember one night I was sitting in our living room watching TV and Lynne was in the kitchen, all of a sudden a programme I had filmed came on, it was just a small part with me playing a doctor on the Bill or something. I only had one line but it was still a buzz that I was on TV. I called out to Lynne to come and have a look, she called back that she was busy. When I went to talk to her later she said that to her being on TV was my job and asking her to come in and look when I was on was like asking her to look at a hole I had just dug if I had been a road digger. That is how she saw my being on screen. I am sure she did not mean it the way it sounded but that moment was a turning point for me and I was hurt. How could something which had taken me years of struggle to even break into and which meant so much to me, mean so little to her. What I could not see at the time was that Lynne saw the industry as a threat to her and to us. That is why she acted that way (and she was right). I found myself longing for someone who felt about the industry as I did, how could I marry someone who looked on acting in the same vein as digging holes? I had no idea what the future had in store for the both of us, only time would tell.

The Bodyguard

I was not really sure when my acting career would really go anywhere so I delved into some other lines of work which made use of my martial arts background, one being that of the bodyguard.

I had looked after celebrities during my time with the stunt team and also looked after members of the Star Trek cast, but this was something quite different. I did a bill paying walk on job on the TV soap Eastenders, and during the shoot I got talking to a chap who I will just call Ian. During a long break in filming he saw me going through some stretching exercises and so he asked if I was a dancer, this led to my telling him about my martial arts background and showing him a few moves, Ian seemed really interested and offered more questions. The result of our conversation was that he eventually opened up to me, he told me that he ran a security organisation which offered close protection to many people the world over and supplied top bodyguards mainly from the military, he said he only did walk on work for a bit of fun. Then he produced an impressive looking security card which seemed to bear out his story. I was intrigued as our conversation became more intense; Ian asked me if I had ever handled a gun. I said yes as part of my stunt training I had fired many guns. With that he asked if I would like to work for him as a bodyguard. I would have to pass an interview and evaluation but with all of my martial arts and weapons training, add to that my past close security experience, he did not think I would have a problem. The action man in me said yes right away. He told me that if accepted I would be assigned to looking after an Arab Prince and his family, I thought wow this sounds like heavy stuff.

When I got home and told Lynne she was not happy about my doing the work, but I saw it as yet another challenge I could not back away from. When the time came I went to London for the interview which was quite in depth, I also had to produce all of my martial arts qualifications. The interview went well and I was offered work right away, a three week contract to be part of a team looking after an Arab Sheik and his family in London. I was given an address and a timetable of my shifts and I was set to start.

A week later I arrived at an exclusive address in London which from the outside looked like a long row of white marble pillared houses, but when I walked through the front door and into the reception area I was shocked to see that the whole row of houses had been knocked through into one long palace like building, complete with a gigantic indoor swimming pool. I was introduced to the head of security who was dressed in a suit and tie (as were we all) but he had a radio mike attached to his collar which was the first sign that he was not just a well dressed guest. It turned out that all the rest of the eight man team were all ex-military, I was the only one who was not. Some were ex-SAS or Para's, and one guy was from the French Foreign Legion, they were not all big guys, but if you looked in their eyes you could see that they had been there. I was shown a firearms locker and a reinforced solid steel safe room where the family would be put in case of an emergency. This introduction did bring home to me that this was a high risk real situation; I would not be dealing with an over affectionate Star Trek fan if things went wrong. My duties were to patrol the garden, vet all the cars in and out of the front gates, and go with the family on trips to Harrods or other places they wanted to visit. I was instructed not to talk to any of the family members unless we were spoken to first except to say good morning. We ate what the family ate which was always food from a massive menu, every breakfast, lunch, dinner and supper had a choice of about six courses, we ate very well but I could not get over all the wasted food, I had grown up with next to nothing, mum working all hours just to feed us, so all of this seemed so unjust somehow.

The guys I worked with were ok for the most part but I knew a couple of them looked at me with doubt as if to say, he's not ex-army so what is he doing here. I kept myself to myself mostly and I can only remember one occasion when one of them said to me, "what would you do if I put one on ya?" (he meant if he punched me). I looked him in the eye and said in my coldest voice, "I think the word you missed was (tried) to put one on ya". I just stood there ready; he paused for a moment, smiled and said, "You're ok mate", and then walked off. The one person I really did not like was the guy from the Foreign Legion, he told us that he always carried an electric stunner with him and that one day he passed a homeless man in the underground who put out his hand and asked for money, the Legion guy said, "I told him ok mate this is for you and pressed my stunner right into his hand, the fucker jumped about three foot in the air then went out like a light". I was always the first to help out genuine people in need, and this creep was against all I stood for. I hated him after that.

The brief I had been given was that the family were at high risk of kidnap because of their wealth and there also could be a possibility of an assassination attempt on the Sheik or his wife, so as you can imagine you could never relax. I used to stand sometimes for ten hours just watching the high garden wall at the back of the house and thinking to myself, if I relax now this could be the one moment someone comes flying over the wall, so it was very draining. You could never take for granted that nothing was going to happen, it was our job to keep these people safe and be ready. The stress was at its worst when going out in public with the family. Four of us would literally surround them at all times. I began to get a good insight into how I felt about the job when one morning the Sheik walked in and I said "good morning sir", he looked right through me as if I did not exist, then it hit me that I might be called upon to risk my life for people who looked on me just as they look on all the food they wasted. They did not value it because they could always afford more; I was just a disposable commodity. I know I would have stepped in front of someone with a gun to save a person I cared about because they were worth it, but I could not honestly say that after that incident I would have risked my life for the Sheik. So at the end of the three week contract I picked up my money and said I would not be back. Another downside of the job was that when I did come home between shifts I could not turn off the grim bodyguard persona I had forced myself to have, that life was not for me.

Affairs Of The Heart

After my bodyguard stint life returned to normality, teaching, the odd walk on part and home life with Lynne. She was lovely as always and content to have me by her side again but I was no longer sure how I felt about us. To be honest looking back on it now I was unsure how I felt about me. I still loved her but I did not know if I was still in love. I had always dreaded the so called normal life, I had mountains which I needed to climb, things I needed to prove to the world and to myself. But Lynne was still a great support and as far as the martial arts were concerned she was behind me 100%. My Jeet Kune Do instructor Richard Bustillo was going to come over from LA to do a seminar for me (his first one in England) which was a massive organisational test, but with Lynne putting together the flyers and handling the bookings for me we pulled it off, the icing on the cake was to have Richard staying with us in our home (one of Bruce Lee's best friends) that was the first of many seminars I would host with sifu Bustillo.

One day I had a fateful phone call from my agent Marcelle which set in motion something that would eventually bring about the end of me and Lynne. The call was for me to work on a TV series called Lovejoy which was to be filmed in Kent, and during the shoot one of the scenes called for me to have a slow dance with an attractive young actress called Carol. Now it sounds like a film script but it really was one of those times. The first time our eyes met and the first time we touched for our on screen dance I knew I had a problem; I fell like a sack of bricks. Like actors tend to do at the end of a shoot a few of us exchanged numbers and addresses, I gave Carol my mum and dad's address in London and dared to hope, part of me hoped I would never hear from her again because I knew I would not be able to help myself, but a bigger part of me hoped I would.

A couple of weeks passed and I had a call from my mum saying I had received a letter. I went on a visit to my parents and picked it up, it was from Carol. She said some lovely things in the letter and suggested we meet up in London, this we did and eventually it happened. We began an affair and at the time we had no idea where it would lead, but we did know it was something very real, we had fallen in love. I still loved Lynne but at that time the butterflies inside me were all caused by Carol.

I was living with my fiancé and my friend who I owed so much to, but I had fallen for an actress who seemed to understand how I felt about the industry and wanted the life I wanted, she had the same dreams I had. I felt guilty doing what I was doing but I began to live a double life, Carol knew about Lynne but I could never let Lynne know about Carol, all I could do was follow my heart and tear myself apart inside for doing so. All of the strain and guilt I began to feel and go through started to have a physical manifestation on me. It almost sounds funny now but I began to be plagued by an itch right up my rear end, it would itch and so I would scratch which caused it to burn and become inflamed and itch so I would scratch, it was a vicious circle (pardon the pun). It would keep me awake at night and if I did fall to sleep I would wake myself up clawing at my backside. I even started to go to bed wearing boxing gloves to stop this happening. It grew worse and worse till the itching and burning began to drive me mad, what with little or no sleep and the constant burning itch, I did not know what to do. It finally came to a head when I was away in Brighton again filming Lovejoy. I was booked into a hotel for the night and woke up about one in the morning in terrible burning agony from my backside. I had clawed myself in my sleep but this time I had somehow scratched up inside myself and I knew I had caused some damage. I checked myself out of the hotel in the middle of the night and I could hardly keep still with the pain. I had no means of transport to get home so I had to ring Lynne. As always she did not let me down, within the hour she was picking me up from Brighton and whizzing me home.

As soon as it was open I rushed to the doctors to be seen as an emergency appointment. Before he examined me the doctor asked if I had undergone any anal sex recently, with this I reacted indignantly and proclaimed, "I am not gay,

I am engaged, to a woman". He gave me a thorough internal examination and sent me for tests to the hospital. It turned out that I had torn some nerves just inside my back passage while scratching, hence the terrible pain, but there was no reason for my itching other than it possibly being stress related. It did eventually subside and I realised that maybe it was the price I paid for betraying someone who never should have been betrayed. In a way I deserved all I got.

Bad Signs

A really great chance for my career happened after yet another call From Marcelle, I had been offered a reoccurring small part as a character named Patrick on a top BBC comedy series called The Brittas Empire. The series starred Chris Barrie of Red Dwarf fame and later the Lara Croft films, the show was to be filmed on location in a town called Ringwood (near Bournemouth) and then at the BBC centre in London, the series turned out to be the best thing I had done to that point. I got on very well with all of the cast and we had a great time, my part on Brittas was to last nearly five seasons. On a couple of occasions when we filmed in front of a live audience at the BBC I got my lovely mum tickets to come and see us film, I would have loved it if my dad could have joined her but he was not really into social gatherings in those days, he was content to be happy for the two of us and hear all the stories later. After the show I took mum up into the BBC bar where she met all the cast and saw loads of other famous TV people, to see her sitting there with that smile of pride on her face meant the world to me, although life had taken me away from time to time mum and dad were still my priority.

As always I continued to visit my parents every chance I got and when I was filming in London and had an early call I would always stay with them. On one of my visits mum said to me that she had noticed a change in my dad, he had not gone for his usual daily walks and had seemed a bit withdrawn so I made it my job to sit down and have a talk with him. Harry did seem different, something in his face had changed somehow, but I couldn't quite put my finger on it and I could also see that he had lost some weight. My poor dad had been through so much during the years that it was hard to get a consistent idea of how he was supposed to be, but during the past couple of years he had been at his best, my dad as he would have been without all the years of illness. I agreed with mum that we would keep a close watch on him and that I would phone every day to see how he was.

As the weeks went by it became very clear that something was wrong, every time I saw him he looked worse, mum had told me that he was eating next to nothing and weight was just falling off of him. So one night mum tried to get to the bottom of why he would not eat and out of the blue he told her, apart from bread and water any other food turned to poison in his body. This news was like a punch in the face, surely after all this time that bastard illness could not be claiming him again; I had to know for sure so I tried to have a father and son talk with him. It had only been during the last couple of years that we had been able to sit and share all the things a father and son should share, I could not bare the thought that we were going to lose all of that again. But no matter what I said he would not listen, the other side of Harry had at long last broken his silence and was again the only voice my dad could hear. My father must have weighed about eight stone by now and for a grown man that was nothing. I spoke to mum and we reluctantly agreed, we had to get him into hospital somehow before he starved himself to death. Both mum and I felt kind of defeated somehow, like we had come through all the storms and just when we thought the sun would last forever we had been struck by a bolt of lightning. It had been many years now since my dad had been into a mental hospital like Cain Hill and in the intervening years they had all been closed down, (thank God) but for his sake we had to do something, (we had been down this road before, many times). I felt terrible doing it but I persuaded dad to come with my mum and I to a hospital called Guys not too far away from our old home. I said to dad that I would get him some help so he would be able to eat again, he looked me in the eye and said, "Ok boy", but I think in his heart he knew, I just hoped he could forgive me. I had phoned ahead to Guys and was initially met with a lot of resistance to my bringing my father in, but I would not take no for an answer, and so the three of us got into a taxi and headed over to London Bridge and Guys hospital.

When we arrived we were shown into a large almost empty room, with only a couple of chairs and a large mirror on the wall, mum and I both sat holding dad's hands to reassure him because we knew of his dread for hospitals, (who could blame him). Five, ten , fifteen minutes went by, I knew what was happening so I stood up went over to the big mirror and smiling into it said, "I know you are watching us from behind this mirror, don't you think it is about time you came and spoke to us". Two minutes later a doctor appeared with a smile across his face and introduced himself to us, then said to me, "that was very astute of you to know about the mirror", I looked right at him and said "let's get something straight, we have been dealing with situations like this for over thirty years, I love my father and my mother loves her husband, we have only brought him here as a last resort to save his life, not to get him locked away just because we feel like it". The doctor then agreed that they had been watching us to see how we treated Harry, to make sure we were there for the right reasons, he could now see we were. Mum and I were then interviewed separately before they spoke to my dad. After speaking to him they agreed he should be admitted right away. They gave us some time alone with him which we filled with hugs, then I looked into my dad's sad eyes held his hand and said, "You know in your heart you need to be in here so you can get well, and to stop poor mum worrying about you so much". He looked at me with resignation and tiredness on his face and just said, "I know boy, I know." We left the hospital without Harry and with my mum in tears. I felt so confused and sad, on one hand I felt relieved he was in a place where he could be helped, but the other part of me felt terrible that he was again back in the place he hated and for the first time it was me, the one he trusted most in the whole world who had put him there.

The Lost Boys

During all of the sad goings on with my dad I had continued to teach at my school, and I have known through many years of study and self examination that by helping people fight their demons you help to fight your own, that was a big part of my martial arts teachings. The first person I ever took under my wing to try and improve his life through training was Alan Knight, who I nicknamed Grasshopper (after the lead character in the old Kung Fu series). When I first started to visit my sister soon after she moved to Plaxtol she began to tell me about this poor skinny boy with buck teeth who used to come and tend her garden and also do odd jobs for her. Sue said she had felt sorry for him because of the home life he had so she had told him about her little Kung Fu brother. Sue said I just had to meet him. When I eventually moved down to live with my sister I finally met Alan and agreed to train him in the martial arts. Alan lived not far from our house and he was the epitome of a downtrodden soul with no self confidence (and I should know all about that) I was in the process of breaking out of that mould myself. He began to confide in me and told me that his father had bullied the family all their life and Alan was afraid of him. I promised that one day that feeling would be a thing of the past.

We ended up training together on and off for about ten years and Alan became a very good martial artist and a confident human being. One day

Alan's dad went for his mother and Alan stepped in between them, he was forced to threaten his father which he did not want to do, but on that day the bullying of the family ended. Alan was the first of what I have come to call the lost boys.

A couple of years later I was at a Star Trek convention and I saw a skinny guy with glasses walking along holding a pair of Nunchaku (clubs joined by chains) martial arts weapons and he had a little gang of people following him. I could not resist it so I went up to him and said, "Excuse me mate can I have a look at your Nunchak's". He smiled and said "ok but don't hurt your self sonny". I took them and whirled them all about my body as I had been trained to do and he just stood there with his mouth open wide. When I finished and handed them back to him he just said "Fucking hell". Martin had been able to use the Nunchaku quite well and used to show people (hence the little group) and he loved the martial arts and Star Trek. This meeting began yet another Grasshopper relationship for me, with my training Martin for many years to come. He had an unfortunate background not unlike mine and he had never had a job, also his life at that time was not great and he did not have a lot to look forward to. We became fast friends as well as teacher student, and over the years I was able to help give him a lot of life lessons and confidence as well as martial arts training. He went on to first being a top martial arts instructor then in later years the head of a company called Men in Black who did loads of weird and wonderful things, and many of the people he employed were formally from unfortunate backgrounds with little or no hope in life. Martin did for them what I helped do for him, and the cycle continues.

Another prime example of helping through training was when I met a young guy named Eric. He came to my martial arts school one day many years after the Alan era and asked for private tuition, I could see from the way he stood, the way he looked, and the nervous twitches and habits that he needed so much more than just the physical side of martial arts training, he reminded me so much of someone, Me, how I used to be during our darkest times. Part of my teaching method is to get to know the person I am training, really get to know their inner self, and it was not long before Eric began to open up to me. His mother suffered from (you guessed it) schizophrenia the dreaded illness which had blighted my life through my father, as it was doing to Eric through his mum. I found a big part of my salvation through the martial arts and here was Eric years later turning to me for the same reasons. Eric lived with his mum who at that time was going through terrible stages of paranoia, and Eric also had a brother George who was all but crippled by eczema all over his body. Eric was a carer with few friends and little hope for the future. As our training began and our relationship developed I took it upon myself to be there for him. I began to open up and tell him that this fit strong martial arts instructor, actor and stuntman, used to be just like him in so many ways, and that if he just found it within himself to get through till tomorrow he could follow his dreams too.

On some days our lessons would just be Eric talking to me as tears streamed down his face; I was his mentor and also his friend. I felt not only for Eric but for his brother I knew he cared so much about so one Christmas I went to a hospital with Eric to visit his brother George who was bedridden and covered from head to toe in bandages, another lonely shy person with the weight of the world on his shoulders. I did my best to lift his spirits too. I know our time training and talking together helped Eric through some of his dark times and even though we lost touch for some years he is now back in touch with me again, older stronger but still battling those inner demons and still looking after his mum, but he has come a long way, he now teaches on the open University and these days he smiles a little more. I am kind of proud of him.

I mentioned early on in this book that I have a kind of Peter Pan complex, never wanting to fully grow up. I also collect figures of Pan. Well the connection goes further because like him I have my own set of lost boys, (and girls) as I call them; people like Eric who needed somebody to help them through. In my martial arts school I do not just teach how to kick ass, I teach and help people to survive life. As well as some really fit strong martial artists I also have some people who life has dealt a rough hand to, such as two brothers (Dave and John) who some people just looked upon as someone to laugh at. I took them under my wing and in spite of their physical and other problems they trained hard and can now hold their heads high and are part of our extended family, they have survived where many others would have fallen by the wayside. We also have a man (Pete) who sometimes visits us, Pete is in his mid seventies and you can tell just by looking in his lovely old eyes that life has been so hard on him, and now he has no one in the world. But bless him he has the face of an angel and the spirit of a lion, and we are his friends now. He came into my school with a little round chap about five foot tall (Dave) they had met in a home and helped each other, Dave joined my club with Pete (free of charge of course) and although he could not hurt a fly he is now no longer alone. Another asset to my club is a really bright young Asian chap (Ajay) who is a computer wizard but he also carries the burden of being a carer for his mother who is yet another sufferer of schizophrenia. Lastly I also train two lovely ladies, Rita, an Asian girl and Michelle a white girl who both suffered the curse of having schizophrenic mothers and fight the demons of the past. We all try to get together once a year for our club Christmas dinner and I make sure that all of my lost boys and girls feel they are part of a family who cares.

The Last Trek

For months Lynne and I continued to make regular trips from Kent to London so we could join mum and support her as she visited dad in hospital, which seemed to be something she had done most of her adult life. He was in a ward for disturbed people, not a mental ward as such but it was a locked door environment none the less. It was so sad to see him back in a hospital again especially now that he was in his sixties (mum too). One day I had a call out of the blue from Richard Arnold, my friend in Hollywood who worked with Gene Roddenberry, he told me that Gene had been very ill too, but unlike my father Gene was physically ill, he invited me to come over for a visit. They were filming Star Trek VI which was to be the last film with the original cast and there was also to be a ceremony in Paramount to honour Gene by dedicating a building to him. I owed Gene a lot for the inspiration he had given me and for all the interest he had shown in a normal poor boy from the Elephant, it would also be the last chance for me to be with all of the original heroes from Star Trek who had adorned the walls of my Star Trek room for so many years, some of whom had even become friends of mine. I felt I had to go, but looking back on it now I never should have done with my father in that condition but I really felt that Harry was in a safe place and mum was relieved knowing he was in good hands so I decided to go back to LA.

It was a shame that Lynne could not come with me but not being self employed as I was getting time off of work was a problem. Before I went to the States I asked for a meeting with the doctor to talk about my dad and his future so he agreed. At the meeting the doctor told me that my father was not responding to medication and was still refusing to eat, so they were considering electric shock treatment, I went through the roof, I explained that my dad had been given dozens of shock treatments over the years, usually because of his extreme symptoms, one course had been for not eating but that was when he was a much younger man, now he was in his mid sixties and was weak from his weight loss, I did not want him given any shock therapy and I made that clear. My dad had told me how they used to strap him to a bed and put a rubber clamp in his mouth before the treatment began, I do not know how much sedation they used in those days but he told me he used to feel the electric crash through his body and lift him off of the table. I know times had changed and the shock treatment was no longer the terrible ordeal it once was but I still wanted none of it for him, he had had enough.

I went to the States knowing in my heart the timing was wrong but I selfishly went anyway hoping for the best. When I got to the States I visited the set of Star Trek VI "The Undiscovered Country", where I met my celebrity friends, Walter Koenig (Chekov) George Takei (Sulu) and Jimmy Doohan (Scotty), I had lunch with Walter and George in the studio then went with Richard Arnold to see Gene. Gene was now walking very slowly with a walking stick after his illness which had been a stroke, but he still remembered me. The last thing he said to me was I am very glad that you liked my show, with that he put his hand on my shoulder and gave me a squeeze, then with the widest of smiles he turned and slowly walked away. That turned out to be the last time I would ever talk to the Great Bird of the Galaxy (his nick name) as he sadly passed away just a few short weeks later, the end of a legend, and of an era. While I was in LA I also visited my Jeet Kune Do instructor Richard Bustillo who insisted I trained with him before I went home. My two passions still existed side by side.

Music No More

As soon as I returned home I went straight to London to see mum, right away I knew something was wrong, she seemed really upset and said that in the two weeks I had been gone dad had changed dramatically. At the end of the first week after I had left the doctors had asked to see mum and had told her that Harry was now in danger of starving himself to death so the choice was being taken out of her hands; they then proceeded to give my dad shock treatment.

After the treatment they had moved him to a smaller hospital which specialised in all kinds of mental disorders but not the horrific places of years ago. I was really upset and angry that all this had happened while I was away, but I rationalised that the doctors had done it for his own good, and surely they knew best? Right away I went with mum to see my father at the new smaller hospital. I was pleased to hear that patients had their own rooms which I thought must be better for a private man like Harry. I really wanted to see dad because a part of me felt guilty for leaving him when I did, but my eagerness to see him soon turned to shock. As I walked in his room I saw my dad sitting on his bed, I stood in the doorway and called to him, when he saw me he did not get up to give me a hug as he had always done on visits, so I walked over to him, bent down and gave him his hug, when I looked into his eyes he seemed to have a kind of permanent wide eyed stare as if he had been surprised and the expression had stayed with him, I held his hand and I could feel it shaking, when I let it go the tremor continued. It was too late for me to rant at any doctors, it was done and my dad had survived, but at what price.

I stayed in London that night so I could visit him again the next day but when we got there, for the first time in our lives my father called out, "no, go, I don't want to see you, go". We were stunned but we did not want to upset him anymore so we left. As we walked out tears ran down my mum's face and I felt as if someone was choking me, but I could not cry for her sake. I had to go back to my home in Kent, the trip to LA had drained away any savings I had so it was time to knuckle back down to work in my martial arts school, it was also time I gave my agent (Marcelle) a call to see if she could drum up some film work. The worry over my dad was a strain but so was the situation I had put myself in with Carol and Lynne. Carol was pressuring me to spend more time with her and Lynne was doing all she could to save our relationship which she knew was in trouble. It had been a long time since Lynne and I had slept together (through my choice) and that alone was breaking her heart, I did not know how much longer I could keep this up, the guilt was tearing me apart and I was starting to hate myself. Around this time in my life I had seemed to make so many wrong decisions, I had selfishly gone to LA when mum and dad needed me and I had gone at a time when Lynne was full of doubt and pain about our future.

As the weeks went on my dad began to grow a little stronger but his shaking hand grew worse, thankfully the episode of him calling for us to go never reoccurred, but something was definitely wrong. Harry started to say strange things and he would sometimes call me by another name! The penny only really dropped when dad came home for a weekend visit. I had brought him an electric organ a couple of years before and he loved it, he would play for hours and record himself singing on it. On this first weekend back home I set the organ up for him and we sat down to listen. When he began to play it sounded as if a chimpanzee had got hold of it and was just slapping his hands up and down over the keys, mum and I were shocked and devastated but we dare not let dad see, after all those years of being a brilliant pianist he could no longer play a note. When we took him back to the hospital and told the doctors they immediately gave him a brain scan and to our horror it showed that he had what they described as an abnormality, further tests was to show that he was in the early stages of Alzheimer's, my father had come through all those years of mental illness to be struck by that other bastard disease. I was sure the last set of electric shock treatment had been a bridge too far and had brought on the Alzheimer's but I had no way of proving it, and the damage was already done.

We began to notice that my dad's face had started to change. He began to develop a kind of mask which had a kind of expressionless expression, except when you made him smile you could still see his eyes smile. Mum being the woman she was, she said she wanted to look after him at home. So the doctors agreed and Harry came home to 27 Oswin Street so his Maggie could look after him.

As always mum was fantastic and she did look after him, she had her pension and an allowance for dad but it was still not much, so every now and then I would have to force money on her, because as I have stated earlier it was the hardest thing in the world for mum to accept help from anyone, even from me. As time passed mum would phone me with stories of dad getting worse, like putting his shoes in the oven, turning the gas on without lighting it, flooding everywhere by leaving the tap on, and even wetting himself sometimes thinking he was on the toilet. I began to see this life taking its toll on mum so unfortunately after a few months Harry had to be taken back into hospital as a live-in patient, he just needed too much care to ever live at home again. But mum, bless her, would not be parted from him so she went through the process of becoming a full time carer with the hospital and went every day to look after dad as well as some of the other patients. I made sure I got to the hospital whenever I could and I even did a live costume stunt show on an open day to raise money for them. I remember dad in the front row during the show telling people that's my boy. Even in his condition he still felt pride in me which was worth a Kings ransom.

You Always Hurt

As I have said, on top of my father's illness the situation with Lynne and Carol was also taking a toll on me. I loved Lynne and my house and my cats, we had seven years together to look back on and she was also my friend,...but I loved Carol in a different way, I had fallen in love with her, we shared the same goals and dreams about the acting profession, she had joined the Elliot agency and Marcelle got us work together all the time. Carol even worked on a couple of episodes of the Brittas Empire with me and people on film sets began to see us as a couple. I even asked mum if Carol could stay in London with her while she looked for a place to live. They got to know one another and I knew that I had forced mum into the same situation, I had put mum between a rock and a hard place. She loved Lynne and thought she would one day be her daughter in law, but mum also saw how I felt about Carol.

I am not sure what would have happened if my hand had not been forced, but it was. One day I had been visiting mum, dad and Carol in London and I decided to show Carol what Kent looked like. I was going to show her around Tonbridge where my friend Glen lived, all have tea back at Glen's then put Carol back on the train home before returning to Lynne, or so I thought. Lynne had known I worked with this girl called Carol and she had often asked me was their anything between us but I had always said no and laughed it off.

On this day after my visit to her, my mum had not realised Carol would be coming back to Kent with me and Lynne had phoned just after I had left to see what train I would be on. Mum had innocently told her and Lynne had decided to meet me at the station to come and see Glen with me. When the train pulled in Carol and I got off and began to stroll along the station hand in hand like any other couple, I looked up just in time to see Lynne making a lunge for Carol. I just intercepted her and managed to grab hold of her as Carol staggered away in shock. I spun Lynne around and pinned her against a wall shouting for her to leave Carol alone. At that moment I had made a choice, I had gone against Lynne to defend Carol, and Lynne was in the right. We had a shouting struggling scene in full view of everyone on the station. I at last got Lynne to agree to go home and finished by saying that I would come home later and explain everything to her. Lynne stormed off leaving Carol shaking and me feeling sick as a dog. I took Carol to Glen's house and tried to calm down before he drove me home to face the music. As we drove I felt like the world was spinning way too fast, I had dreaded this moment, and here it was.

When I got home Lynne was waiting stony faced and she came right out with it; "are you having an affair with Carol?" All I could say was, yes. With that word my poor lovely Lynne exploded, she came at me swinging, and after all of my years of training no one could hit me if I did not want them to, but I just stood there and took it. It was the beginning of the end, I was guilty as hell, I had betrayed our love. After what seemed forever things calmed down and all we could both do was stand and cry.

It did not happen right away and a couple of weeks later Lynne even told me she still loved me, but as the saying goes, you can't tread twice on the same piece of water. I know it broke her heart and to be honest it broke mine too, but it was all that I could see to do. I moved out, left my Lynne, my home and my cats. I rented rooms in a house in Tunbridge Wells just a couple of miles from our house and eventually I signed my part of the house over to Lynne, she had put down the deposit but the rest of our home belonged to the both of us. After all I had done to her I wanted nothing of value to take with me, she deserved to keep everything.

I arranged for a friend to bring his small van to the house while Lynne was at work and move all of my clothes and bits out. Looking back now I know that I was to blame for our relationship not working, Lynne was a lovely girl, all any man could want. In my defence all I can think of is that having my teenage years virtually taken away by Harry meant I missed out on so much, and when I found myself in the world of show business I could see all the mountains I wanted to climb, and all the things I wanted to prove to myself and to the world, and I could not do that in Toad Rock with Lynne. I also fooled myself into thinking that only someone in the industry could share my passions and my dreams, how wrong I was. With Lynne it really was the old cliché, the right love at the wrong time, and in my heart I missed her terribly.

As I adjusted to my new life of living in someone else's home again and wrestling with my pangs of guilt, I vowed that all this would be for a reason. I had left Lynne because I had fallen in love with Carol but also because of this drive to succeed in the film industry, and so I reaffirmed to myself I would make it. Mum and dad still had to have a happy ending and it was up to me to make that happen.

The house I moved into was owned by an Iranian chap named Farid who I had met a few years earlier and had happened to bump into again while looking for a place to live. Farid was great to live with and he was glad of my company. I saw a lot of Carol and she began to stay with me during the week, so much so that Farid started asking for more rent money because now there were two of us virtually all of the time.

Every weekend I would visit mum and we would go and see dad, although he had settled into his new life in hospital I did feel so sorry that he had ended up there. I used to sit on his bed with him between my legs and my arms around him watching TV; I had become the one feeling protective of him after all those years of him protecting me. I bought him a video recorder so he could record and watch what he wanted, but one day he got confused and poured a bowl of water on it, goodbye video. Harry was sometimes able to talk about things in his now weak voice, other times he struggled to understand, but he always knew who we were. One day when I was not with her a disturbed patient came into my dad's room and without warning punched mum in the face. Dad who now weighed next to nothing jumped up and shouted "leave my Maggie alone", and shaped up to the much larger and younger man preparing to fight for the woman he still loved. Even with all he was going through and all the things he was forgetting due to his illness, he still knew she was his Maggie.

And So It Ends

The months tumbled by and my fathers birthday was approaching, the people in the ward loved him and with mum's help wanted to throw a party in his honour, it would be a chance for everyone in that sad place to lift their spirits. Unfortunately the day of the party I was due to film on the police series The Bill, it was a small but reoccurring role as a duty solicitor (my name tag read Mr Whitlock). I could not afford to give up the part but I really wanted to be there for my dad. Luckily the filming wrapped by late afternoon so I jumped on a train from Wimbledon where The Bill was filmed and rushed to the hospital, I got there covered in sweat from my frantic trip and hurried up to dad's floor. I think he had given up on seeing me at his party because when I finally walked onto the ward his face actually changed from the masked expression the illness made him wear into a big smile. As I came closer he got up and walked towards me with his arms stretched out in front of him and gave me a hug that I will keep with me forever.

Mum had dressed him in his best shirt and jumper and finished off with a lovely big velvet bow tie he had had for years. I stayed and watched my mum hold my dad for a slow dance to some old record which was playing, and after all they had been through together you could still see the love they so obviously still shared. The time came for me to get back to Kent so I gave them both a big hug before I left, and just before I went out of the door I turned to look back and gave my dad a thumbs up, he lifted his weak arm and did the same to me. That was to be the last happy memory I would ever have of Harry, a few days later I received a call from my sister telling me that dad had suffered a massive seizure of some kind and I had better get to London as quickly as I could. Carol and I dropped everything and jumped in the car. As we sped through Tunbridge Wells I remember seeing an old couple sitting on a bench together holding hands, I said through bitter clenched teeth, that's how my parents should have ended up.

As we walked into the hospital mum came up to me and sobbed in my arms, my sister Sue was also there along with a couple of my dad's sisters. Harry had apparently been sitting on the toilet and had some kind of heart attack or stroke, we were told to expect the worst. Everyone was in and out of dad's room but it was my sister and I who sat with him none stop for eleven hours, my dad was awake for most of the time but was unable to talk and would sometimes just stare at the bottom of the bed as if he could see someone. In those hours when Sue was taking a break I said to him all the things a son could tell his father, mainly that I loved him which was something I had rarely said to him during our lifetime, but he knew I always had, even in the darkest years when I also hated him.

The terrible thing which made those last hours even more painful for us was the fact that every breath my father took was done with a sad low moan and the doctors said they did not know how he was holding on (but that was Harry boy). Midnight came and went and Sue had to head home, and by that time my poor mum looked as if her legs would not hold her up anymore. A doctor said that we should all go home and try and grab some rest because dad was now stable for the night. For mum's sake I thought we should go home for a while, so we all bent down and kissed my dad's forehead saying go to sleep Harry boy we will see you later, dad's eyes were still open but we were not sure if he could see or hear us. Mum was the last one to leave his room and tears rolled down her cheeks as she walked away. We got back to 27 Oswin Street at about one thirty in the morning and as we turned the light on in the living room the phone rang... we all froze. As I picked up the receiver a doctor's voice said "Mr Carrigan, you need to get back here now". Mum just said oh no and sank into a chair with her face in her hands, I said that I would go back alone. Carol drove me to the hospital and I ran up the stairs full of dread, a doctor was waiting for me and I knew by his face. He said he was sorry but my father had passed away just ten minutes ago...Did I want to see him, I said yes. I had never seen a dead person let alone someone who had been such a pivotal part of my life. I am an actor and we have to imagine ourselves in many situations to be able to act accordingly, but I could never have imagined my reaction. As I walked into my dad's room not knowing what to expect or how to react, I looked up and caught my first glimpse of him. I froze at the door in mid stride, I just stood there for what seemed ages and the first thing that came into my mind was, why have they covered him in white powder (stupid I know) my father was sitting up in bed with a frowned expression on his face and he was completely white, I also saw that his fingernails were completely black, his colour was such a shock. I composed myself and walked over to him, stroked his cold forehead and just said, oh dad, I kissed his head, stood there for a moment then walked away. In the car with Carol I was kind of numb, he was gone, Harry was gone, the man, the father who I had loved and at one time hated, the one who had destroyed part of my life but who had also made me who I am was gone, what would our world be like without him in it. When I got back to my old home I walked up those many flights of stairs and into the living room, looked over at my tiny little hero of a mum and said, "He's gone". Then both our worlds erupted into tears that never wanted to stop.

Life After Harry

As the days passed following my fathers passing mum and I got on with handling all the things which needed sorting, the biggest of which was Harry's funeral. My dad always said he hated cremations so he was to be buried in a cemetery in London where all his and my mum's family were. As the time for the funeral drew closer I stepped in more and more to help mum, so did Sue, although it was harder for her living further away. The day came when we all went to see my father lying in his coffin to say goodbye one last time. Now part of the legacy he had left me with was the love of childhood , not my childhood but the idea of never growing up too much, dad always said to me be forever childlike without being childish. A few years ago I had started to take an interest in the concept of the Peter Pan stories and collected some ornaments and figures relating to him I also found a lovely Pan figure badge, so as I said my last goodbye to my father I placed my Pan badge inside his suit lapel, so he would be forever young.

All of dad's brothers and sisters turned up for the funeral, so did my mum's sister Aunt Joan who had also been to see dad in hospital during his last illness. Mum was determined to finally give Harry the recognition he had been denied in life, on this the day of his funeral. So, all of his flowers and wreathes were laid outside of the house in Oswin Street where most of the dramas of dad's life had been played out, and many people came out of their houses to watch as Harry's hearse drew up at no 27.   My old friend Kevin's dad (Jack) used to ask Harry into his house sometimes to play his organ, and they would often end up singing at the top of their voices together, I suppose Jack was the closest thing to a friend my father had in years, so when the funeral procession slowly began to move off down Oswin Street Jack stepped out in front of the funeral car which made it stop, he then bowed his head, waited for a moment and then stepped back onto the pavement.   It was a very moving tribute which I will never forget and still moves me today.   Jack himself has since passed on and no doubt somewhere beyond our hearing the two of them still sing together to their hearts content.

All of my dad's three brothers had done very well in their respective careers, and everyone was dressed in their smart dark suits for the funeral with dad's sisters dressed just as aptly, a somewhat hypocritical gesture considering what little support some of them had been to him in life. As we all stood around the grave and Sue and I supported our sobbing mum the heavens suddenly opened up and it rained as if it would never stop, everyone got soaked, I remember thinking that was Harry boy having the last laugh on all of them.

My uncle and Godfather (Joke), John had given us the use of the pub he owned to hold the after funeral get together, it was the first time I had ever been in his place and there they all stood, dad's brother's Bobby, Danny, and Johnny, recounting stories of when Harry was young, all stories of before he was ill, as if he never existed after his illness began. The only one I had ever really spent time with was dad's youngest brother Danny, who we had not seen a lot of over the years, but when we did see him it always came across that he cared, and Danny always reminded me of my Harry, especially in looks. Bobby was ok but even though I lived in the same house as him for many years, I never really got to know him. Then there was Uncle John. As I stood in his pub beside my girlfriend Carol Johnny came up to us and said, I hear you are budding actors, well I know people who can help get you an Equity card. I took great satisfaction in looking him in the eye and saying "no thanks uncle I have already earned mine".

Coming To Terms

When my father died I really missed him a lot, there was such a hole in my life, I know he put us all through hell in the past but it was not his fault, he did not ask to be given that cruel disease, the real Harry truly was a lovely man. I found it hard to come to terms with the fact that he had seemed to have brought his schizophrenia under control during the last few years and he and mum were just beginning their golden years as the loving couple they had been in the beginning of their relationship, only to be cut down by Alzheimer's. I did and still do believe in God but I could not bring myself to say any prayers at night for over a year.

Following the loss of my dad I was still determined more than ever to make something of myself so that I could give my lovely long suffering mum some kind of a life, free of worry and debt, a life she so deserved. I stayed at home in London with mum to help her through these first few horrible days and to be honest I needed to be with her too, but true to the way her life had gone, fate struck again.

It was not quite two weeks since Harry's funeral and mum had gone to a supermarket at the Elephant and Castle shopping centre to do her weekly shopping, as she bent down to a low vegetable rack a pile of large swedes suddenly came loose from the top shelf and crashed down onto the back of my mothers neck knocking her unconscious. I do not know how long she was out but when she revived they sent someone to walk home with her. I was in the living room and heard someone walking slowly up the stairs, as the door opened I turned to see that it was mum and the sight almost sent me into panic mode. She was as white as a ghost and I could see she could hardly stand, I rushed over to her and sat her down, I immediately wanted to call for an ambulance but mum would not hear of it, she said she just needed to lie down and change her clothes. It turned out that she had wet herself as she lay unconscious. I put her to bed and phoned for an emergency doctor who came out right away. After looking at her he insisted that she go for an x-ray and was good enough to drive her himself. I was fuming at the way my lovely frail looking mum had been treated by the store, they should have called an ambulance right away no matter what my mother said. I grabbed my camera and stormed over to the centre. When I arrived I took pictures of the scene and asked some of the staff just what had happened. After writing everything down I went to meet my mum at the hospital. I was glad to see that she was looking a bit better now and a doctor told me she would be allowed home for complete bed rest with her neck in a collar and loads of pain killers.

Thank God my mum was a strong woman, the life she had led had made her that way but she soon became very unwell as the shock of the accident set in. I was broken hearted for her, as if her life were not already hard enough, I wanted some justice. I contacted a solicitor and he agreed that mum had a very strong case for compensation, thus began months of mum being looked at first by medical doctors on the supermarkets behalf, then she was sent to be evaluated by psychiatric doctors, again on the supermarkets behalf. They almost tried to say that because mum was depressed by the loss of my father, she could have done this herself (what a load of bollocks). She was in her sixties and was quite frail due to the life she had led and the last thing she would do was throw a load of Swedes onto her own head. My mum had shown in the past that no matter how frail her body got she was always so strong in spirit and to resort to a stunt like that was impossible even to think of.

As the months went on she had constant pain at the top of her spine where the impact had been and she began to get pain in her hands and other places over her body, a doctor said the blow to the top of mum's spine had set off the arthritic nerve in her body. Before the accident she used to kick her leg above her head being an ex-acrobat and a dancer, even after her sixtieth birthday, but now parts of her were suddenly freezing up. After months of sometimes humiliating examinations and questions she was awarded three thousand pounds in compensation by the store, which after all she had been through and for all the future pain her neck would give her, was a paltry sum, but mum was just glad to get it over with, and to her three thousand pounds was like three million.

My poor mum had existed for years by having loans from money lenders who she knew (mostly without us knowing) and with dad not being able to work and little money coming in it was the only way she had got all of us through, and little did I know that some of those debts with massive interest still existed. I later found out that mum used some of the money to pay off the long standing loans, but the hardest part was trying to stop her giving any of the money to us. All through her life she had given everything to everyone else and left nothing for herself, but that was and always would be the nature of my lovely mum. It took time for all of us to get used to a world without Harry, but as the saying goes life must go on.

Carol and I wanted to get a place of our own and with my filming on The Bill and The Brittas Empire, as well as all our auditions not to mention mum being in London, it seemed to be the only place to again come back to live. Through an actor friend of Carol's we got to hear about a lovely ground floor flat for rent in Wimbledon (close to where I filmed The Bill) it was also fully furnished so we went for it, and before we knew it we were living back in London. I still had my martial arts school in Kent so it meant that twice a week I still had to go back to the garden of England, which also meant I could have the best of both worlds.

Wimbledon turned out to be a great place to live, and being back in London we had a great social life with all of our actor friends, I could also pop in on mum to make sure she was ok during the week and not have to just wait for weekends. I always wanted to give my mum good experiences and share all I could with her, she had never had the chance to feel like someone special (and she had never asked to) but to me she was the most special and inspirational person I knew so she deserved all I could give her. One Saturday when I was filming the live part of Brittas at the BBC centre I again got my mum tickets to come and see the show being taped as part of the studio audience and after the show I took her up into The BBC bar to met all of the cast and sit with us, she sat there completely out of place but glowing with pride and loving every moment. But I am afraid the hard times for my lovely mum were far from over.

About a year after the supermarket incident I had a call saying that she had been rushed to hospital with terrible vomiting and stomach pains. When I arrived at the hospital she was in the casualty department and she looked terrible, almost as if she was near to death. When I walked in to her cubicle and up to her bed she did not see me so I reached out and took her hand, as I did I said, "I am not letting you go anywhere", with that she seemed to come to life again and told me that I had always been her strength. I called a doctor over and asked what was wrong, he said that as far he could see it could just be a bad case of colic, I could not believe it, she looked so ill; he then said we could take her home. I was not happy with his answer but I knew mum wanted to be out of the hospital. I knew I could not let her be alone like this so Carol and I took her back to Wimbledon with us, but I was so worried because I almost had to carry her back to the car. That night mum had a fitful painful sleep and I stayed up all night watching her. The next day we drove her down to my sisters in Essex so she could be looked after full time, Sue did not have a job so I knew that would be possible. We left mum with Sue and came home knowing mum would be in good loving hands.

Two days later Sue phoned to say mum had been rushed back into hospital (in Essex this time) and they were to give her emergency surgery. They had found out that all the pain and vomiting had been caused by a burst bowel (which the London hospital had missed) and she could have died if they had not discovered it, the angels were with us this time and the operation was a complete success. A happy foot note was that while my mum was recovering at my sisters I had to go away on location to film The Brittas Empire and when the cast got to hear about my mum they all signed a big get well card to her, headed by none other than Mr Brittas himself Chris Barrie. When she was well enough mum returned home to Oswin Street and I made sure that till she was

back to being indestructible Maggie I would watch
her like a hawk.

One Stunt Too Many

As life continued with us all trying to get back to normal I received a call from Martin a former student and friend of mine from Nottingham. Following our years of training together Martin had started his own multi level company, part of that company held two day stunt courses for would be stunt people, like I had first gone on several years ago, only this time I was asked to go along as one of the course trainers. Martin had been involved in many of my live stage and stunt shows in the past and this had planted the seed of an idea in his mind which had led to the courses. I agreed to come and take part mainly because Martin had said the course would be covered by more than one major TV station. I thought it could only do good for my career (and the money would come in handy too), at this time I was still doing the odd film or TV show which used my experience as a stunt performer as well as an actor and I would put myself forward as an action actor. This meant I could play an acting role and also do as many of my own stunts as the director would allow. So off I went prepared to spend a long tough weekend in Nottingham, ready for whatever may come (if only I knew).

The course started off well with myself and Paul Flanagan (a stunt man/actor friend of mine) putting course attendees through screen combat techniques and basic reactions, then two TV stations turned up both at once to film us for the local evening news programmes. The first crew wanted their female reporter to beat Paul and me up on camera (which she did) then they wanted us to demonstrate a screen fight and do some kind of high fall. One guy from the other station then said could you do a stair fall right into the camera. Now we were in massive rooms inside an old building, and the only way to get up to or down from this room was by long flights of stone stairs. Paul and I went to look at the stairs and see if a fall would be possible, I counted twenty one hard stone steps leading up to the stunt room and concluded that I could do a backward role down all them. I had performed many stair falls in the past and part of the secret to avoiding injury (apart from wearing knee elbow and coxic pads) was momentum, become a rolling object with no bits sticking out to get broken, but, (and this was a big but) we saw that at the bottom of the stairs was just a five foot wide landing before a wall, then a left turn to more stairs. I said to Paul that I knew I could do the backwards fall ok but with the speed I would build up I knew I would not be able to stop myself from hitting the wall. He agreed with me and said that it was dangerous, but being me…

The cameras were waiting and the students were waiting (and my ego was waiting) so I said oh what the hell, I will hit the wall but I can take it, my body had been smashed about for years and (pain don't hurt) boy what a bad choice I was about to make. I got into position at the top of the stairs and looked back over my shoulder, it looked a long way down but I had been in these situations with these feelings before so to me it was another chance to challenge myself, to prove myself. So with my heart pounding I launched backwards, I remember rolling over and over really fast, no pain so far and then...nothing. The next thing I remember was coming round in the road outside the building with my head in someone's lap and a TV camera pointing in my face, then in a stupefied half conscious voice I said, did you get the shot. I then insisted on getting to my feet and trying to walk back into the building but my legs buckled under me sitting me back down. Apparently about eight stairs from the end of my role my feet pushed out onto a stair and my body unrolled cannoning the back of my head into the wall just narrowly missing a window ledge (I was so lucky).

When an ambulance came I again insisted on walking up into it with all the cameras from the news stations still rolling, but as soon as the doors closed I just collapsed onto the trolley. I can remember saying to the ambulance man I think I live in Kent with my girlfriend, I did not really know where or even who I was at that moment. I was rushed to hospital for x-rays and they said that thankfully I had not fractured my skull but I did have concussion and needed nine stitches to the back of my head. By the time they released me it was evening and I still felt terrible, but I insisted on going back to tell the people on the course that I was ok and to take what had happened to me as a warning that stunt work was not a game. I spent the rest of the night throwing up every ten minutes which was horrible and I was watched over by a dear friend of mine named Dave Wardale who had come from Liverpool to be with me on the course. It was one of the worst nights I have ever had and I will never forget how Dave helped me get through it. The next day I was put on a train (on my own) back to London with my head feeling like it would drop off, and every now and then I would feel the carriage spin and I would have to stagger to the toilet and throw up.

When the long train journey was eventually over I was met at the station by Carol and as I walked down the platform I was more like a slow moving Zombie than the John she knew. Back at the flat I continued to be sick every few minutes so we went to a hospital because I knew this could not be right. After another set of tests it was found that I had damaged the vegas nerve at the base of my skull. The vegas nerve controls many of our autonomic functions which is why I had been vomiting so much, I had been really lucky the injury could have killed me or at the very least left me with permanent problems. Because my body had been spinning when I hit the wall apparently my brain continued to spin for a fraction after impact, which caused damage to the brain stem. I was given tablets to put under my tongue fifteen minutes before a got up in the morning to stop the sickness until my head stabilised, I had to see the doctor a few more times but he said eventually I should make a full recovery.

It took me quite some time to begin to feel normal again and I began to notice some strange side effects. For a while after the accident I would pause during a conversation to find words that would escape me, and also when reading a script out loud I would misread or mispronounce words a lot, and being an actor this was not a good thing. I also had to work hard to get my writing back to normal, for some reason it seemed to slope off to one side. But the longer lasting effect which still lasts to this day was that I no longer felt invulnerable, I had nearly been killed and that was an eye opener. For a while my confidence in myself took a nose dive and I seemed to want to walk on egg shells. I am now back to my normal boldly go self, but the good thing which came out of that horrible time was that I decided to no longer do stunts on their own, I focused all my attention on my acting. Now if I play a part which requires action I am happy to do all my own fights and falls (if the director allows) but I leave the really big stuff to the real stuntmen.

Mr Star Trek

While I had been recovering from my head smash, my lovely old mum had also been recovering from her operation. She had at last returned home to London and so for a while we kind of kept an eye on each other. Life was hectic with TV work, auditions and my martial arts club in Kent. The more I spoke to people the more it became clearer that there was enough interest for me to open another martial arts club in Wimbledon, so I searched high and low until I found a hall I could teach in during the evenings. As I had done years ago with my first club in Kent I put the word out that I would hold a free demonstration night and all were welcome, suffice to say that I must have wowed them because I had loads of people eager to sign up, which meant I could now open my second school, which was a relief because there was never enough acting work about. As an actor you had to have more than one string to your bow just to survive or sign on the dole, which was something I had never done.

A fortunate break came by way of a phone call from an actor friend of mine who also ran a promotional agency, he said that a company called Bandai had landed a licence to produce Star Trek merchandise and were holding interviews for the London toy fair. They wanted people to talk about and demonstrate all of their new line of Star Trek toys and collectables, preferably someone who knew something about

Star Trek. Well this seemed like a chance tailor made for me. I turned up for the auditions with many other hopefuls but when they heard that I had actually worked on the show and I seemed to know everything about Star Trek that was it. I landed the job as the Bandai resident Trek expert, not only did I do the London toy fair's for several years they also used me as a kind of mini Star Trek celebrity to appear in shops in full Star Trek uniform, sign autographs and promote the line of collectables. They even went a bit over the top and had posters made up for me to sign, it was all great fun and fantastic for the ego. Word somehow began to spread and soon it seemed I was being contacted by every company who had a Star Trek product to promote or had a Trek-tie in. This meant for a long period of time I had none stop work related to Star Trek, the best of which was when a massive exhibition of sets, props and costumes was to go on tour all over England.

The first place the tour went was to Edinburgh in Scotland which is where I had my audition for the tour, and as before I got the job. This time the job involved being in charge of all of the actors employed to be in Trek uniform and man the various sets and exhibits, I also had to hold the auditions and help choose the people who worked as the Trek guides. We also had to host corporate evenings where companies would hire the sets to host their company awards or just for a party, this meant I would have to be in uniform and give many a speech as Captain Kirk, sometimes even as a Klingon. As a tie-in to the exhibitions many TV shows came to the sets or wanted the sets taken to them, one such show was the famous Blue Peter series who wanted to do a Star Trek special. I was asked to help write the script and appear in a short Blue Peter style episode as a Klingon and although it was not working on the real classic Star Trek, for a couple of years it almost felt as if I was. I had become Mr Star Trek and little did I know what influence Star Trek would still have in my future life, just when I needed it most.

Surprise Visitors

One morning out of the blue I had a phone call; it was from Walter Koenig who played Chekov in the original Star Trek series. I had met Walter at conventions but we had only really become friends after we met for lunch one day in LA with Richard Arnold. I had spent a lot of good times with Walter since that day and I had even been to his home, I also knew his wife Judy and his daughter Danielle. We were now firm friends but he was also still one of my childhood heroes. In the call Walter said that he and his son Andrew were in England and had been messed around by the people they were supposed to be staying with and were at their wits end, they needed some friendly faces and a place to stay for a couple of days. I knew Walter could have afforded to stay in any hotel he wanted so I felt really honoured that he had asked to stay with me, I felt honoured and flummoxed at the same time. The thought of Walter Koenig and his son staying in my flat was mind boggling. I of course said yes right away and Carol and I set to preparing for our guests.

When Walter and Andrew finally arrived and we had settled them in Carol showed Andrew around while I sat beside Walter on the sofa, it suddenly occurred to me that this was the first time I had ever been alone with him and he was in my home to boot. As we sat together there was a pregnant silence which Walter picked up on so he turned to me and said, "Buddy if you feel awkward we can stay somewhere else". I then relaxed and came clean saying, "sometimes it's hard separating Walter the friend from the person I used to see with the rest of my heroes plastered all over the walls of my old Star Trek room", I apologised for my awkwardness and we were fine after that. Walter has stayed with me several times since then and I have also stayed at his home in LA. I am proud to say that our relationship has grown into a deep and lasting friendship based on trust and mutual respect, (with just a tad of hero worship).

Something else happened during Walters stay which again almost made me pinch myself, but it was another wonderful moment for me. I had arranged months before for my martial arts instructor Richard Bustillo to come over to England and put on a seminar for me and my students, Richard was supposed to be staying in my flat, but because of Walters unexpected arrival I had been forced to put Richard in a hotel. It turned out that sifu Bustillo and Walter were due to be flying back home the same day so it seemed sensible to take them to the airport together. Up to the day they were due to leave they had not met but on the last day Richard came into my flat and then it happened, two of the biggest influences in my life came together, in front of me shaking hands, an original crew member from Star Trek and one of Bruce Lees best friends, in my front room, wow. During the drive to the airport

Walter asked Richard all about Bruce and Richard asked Walter all about Star Trek, it was unreal.

End Of Oswin

Mum had managed since dad passed away as mum always did, never complaining and never asking for any thing, but I did worry about her living alone at the Elephant and Castle, it was not the place it had been when I was growing up, it had become increasingly threatening to say the least. I am not prejudice in any way but it was a fact that there had been many drug related crimes in the recent past and many muggings. I did not find out till much later that mum had been flashed by a black guy in the subway who had told her to grab hold of this as he flashed his private parts at her. At the time she had been shopping and had a tightly wrapped cabbage in a plastic bag and she had swung this at him shouting, grab this you bastard, her swinging vegetable hit him in the temple which took him by surprise making him lose his footing which gave people a chance to come to her aid as he ran off. I was even more afraid when I also heard that she had been mugged by yet another black man who grabbed her bag and dragged her along the floor because she would not let go of it, luckily she was only slightly hurt, it could have been much worse.

I had often spoken to mum about her moving to somewhere safer but she had always said that she wanted to stay in the place she had been used to all of her life and would only ever move to her beloved Kent (now an impossible dream). I was really surprised when on one of my visits she said to me that she had decided to go and live with my sister in Essex, it surprised me but I was also glad that at last she would be in a safer place and not alone anymore. Mum moving would also spell the end of my family home too because all of my childhood memories were in that house, including all of my childhood toys and my famous Star Trek room, still as I had left it in perfect exhibition condition, complete with my Captain Kirk chair, my shuttlecraft interior and my massive beloved Trek collection.

Mum had already decided with my sister on a moving date so I just had to do something with all my stuff. I was living with Carol in a furnished flat in Wimbledon and I had a display case with my most treasured pieces in, such as, some real props and stuff given to me by Gene Roddenberry but I had nowhere to put the rest of my beloved collection which had helped keep me sane through those long dark years when Harry was at his worst. I had been to a memorabilia show a few weeks before and had spoken to a chap who dealt in collectables, especially Trek collectables and he had given me his card, I gave him a call on the off chance he might be interested in buying a couple of things. So, I arranged for him to come to my mums house the next day.

When the guy eventually arrived and walked into my room his jaw just fell open, he said I had the biggest Star Trek collection he had ever seen and would like to buy all I could offer him, he also said he knew it was worth a lot of money, probably more than he could pay. I was between a rock and a hard place and time was against us. In the end he offered me fifteen hundred pounds (I had looked my collectables up and they were worth many hundreds of pounds more) and I had to except. He also saw my father's piano which Harry had loved so much and had been his only escape from the pain of his illness. We let the piano go for two hundred pounds but the chap promised that he wanted it for his family, not to sell it, and that he would give it a good home, so we agreed.

My Star Trek room had been my refuge, my friend and my escape from all the madness which literally was the other side of Harry, it had meant a lot to me in my life for so long, so before I was forced to dismantle and lose it forever I cleaned and dusted everything in the room and filmed it all on video one last time complete with music and a narration. When the collection had finally been boxed up and taken away along with my fathers piano I walked back into my now nearly empty room, took a couple of buttons from my Captain Kirk chair to keep for old times sake and with a lump in my throat smashed up the chair along with my shuttlecraft. If only I could have found a way to preserve them, but it was too late now my room was no more.

In the days to follow as I helped my mum pack she reluctantly told me one of the reasons she had finally decided to leave Oswin Street. Uncle Bob and his wife Jennifer who lived in the lower part of the house and had owned the property for some years now, had apparently brought a man in to inspect the top floors where my parents lived, this had happened a couple of years ago while my dad was still with us and living upstairs with mum. They had come up to inspect the rooms for reasons we could only guess at, but after his viewing the chap had said that with no hot water or bathroom and with damp everywhere no more rent could be charged for the rooms. After Harry had died mum had started to feel under pressure, she knew that the house was in a very sought after location and many of the houses in the road were being extended or renovated for new well off city people, but with mum being what was called, a sitting tenant, my aunt and uncle would not be able to do anything like selling the property unless they sold the house with her in it.

One day Jennifer had gone up to my mum and said, I am going to have all of your rooms renovated and hot water put in and maybe even a bathroom, so you will have to move out for a while. Now this could have been seen as a kind move by Jennifer or something else, but whatever it was my mother did not take it lying down and they had a blazing row. My mum was on her own, still with all the pains and problems from her hiatus hernia, her neck giving her a lot of pain from her supermarket accident, she was still not fully recovered from her burst bowel operation and she obviously still had all the pain inside from losing her Harry, now Jennifer drops this bomb on her. Jennifer and my dad's brother Bobby owned the house, so mum was not really in a good position to argue. She had lived upstairs all those years and no one had bothered to help her out before, so why now? This is just my opinion, but if this was an offer of help, they were going about it the wrong way. On the day mum left 27 Oswin Street I went with her and said goodbye to all the memories good and bad which dwelled there and we both said farewell to an era which had to be lived to be believed.

Join The Legion

I had been in some good film and TV productions over the years with a couple of good small parts, I had even written, produced and acted in my own film called The Need. I filmed it over a two year period and it cost me about £8000, and for my first attempt at producing a movie it turned out very well, but in trying to get it out for all to see I had been taken for a ride by a distribution company which ended up costing me more money and The Need languishing on a shelf collecting dust so I was still desperate for (as we say) that big break.

One day Carol was looking through a casting list of all current and planned productions in a mail out you could pay for called PCR, she called me over and said she had spotted something. It was a planned sci-fi pilot which was going to be shot called Legion and they wanted actors who also must be proficient in the martial arts, I thought this could be the one, so I sent my CV photo's and show reel to the production address. A few days later I received a phone call from the writer/producer of the show (Neil Jackson) who said he was very impressed with what I had sent him and would like me to go to Birmingham for a meeting. I was over the moon and danced all over the living room (it's an actor thing). This show sounded just perfect for me, so high ho, high ho it's off to Birmingham I go.

At the meeting I made sure I showed Neil (the writer/producer) all I could bring to the production and at the conclusion of the interview he offered me one of the lead roles in the series (wow) at last. As the weeks went on I had more meetings with Neil and became more and more involved in the series pre production. When Neil listened to all of my suggestions and heard that I had produced my own film he offered me the additional role of associate producer. I jumped at the chance and began by helping to gather the rest of the cast together which included my actress girlfriend Carol, not just because she was my girlfriend but because she was a good actress. The weeks went by and I helped audition many of the cast members mostly unknown hungry actors, the last person I contacted was my friend from the original Star Trek cast Walter Koenig. I sent Walter the script (which he liked) and soon we had our star on board.

I was due to be a guest at a big Star Trek convention alongside some very big names from the world of sci-fi so I suggested to Neil that the con would be a great place to launch Legion to the fan community, we put together a short promo tape including some great concept visuals of what the show would look like and I took to the stage in front of 1.500 people. I did my usual talk about my past career and my involvement with Star Trek and Gene Roddenberry, told some funny stories from productions I had been on and ended my show by taking charity donations to kick a stunt bottle off of a fans head on stage, this went down really well and raised quite a bit of money for the charity. Before I left the stage I talked briefly about Legion before introducing its creator Neil Jackson, as part on Neil's presentation he introduced all the new cast of Legion up on stage (apart from Walter who was in LA) and the crowd reacted really warmly, they seemed hungry for some gritty British sci-fi. After the great successful launch on stage a friend of mine (Tom) helped me organise a champagne reception in one of the hotel function rooms so all the cast and crew of Legion could meet together for the first time. Two of my fellow convention guests also turned up because they were interested in joining the show, (Mark Ryan) from a TV series called Robin of Sherwood and (Robin Curtis) an actress who had been in two of the Star Trek movies. Although we did not know who he was at the time a TV producer/director (Barry) had been in the audience and chose to join our get together, the reception was a really good idea and let all the cast and crew really get to know each other. Mark and Robin let it be known that they would also like to be considered for a part in Legion and Neil had no hesitation in signing them up right away and the new director guy Barry offered his services and jumped on board too. Barry seemed to go out of his way to sing my praises and spent the whole reception talking to me which was fine because from what I heard he was a good producer/director and in this business you can never know too many of those.

After the con Barry and I met up first for lunch and then dinner which progressed to him visiting Carol and I at the flat, we all felt that a friendship had begun. Now I do not quite understand how it happened but the next I knew Barry had somehow bought all the rights to Legion from Neil Jackson. He then proceeded to replace all of the cast which had been assembled, except Walter, Mark, Robin and to our great surprise Carol and I. One new cast member was added to our ranks, Jason Connery (son of Sean) who was a friend of Marks from his Robin of Sherwood days, (Jason had been Robin). I felt really sorry for all of the cast who had been so suddenly dropped from the production but the term cut throat business was not far wrong. After all of these goings on Barry became even closer to Carol and I (from his side anyway) and would often come to our flat for dinner and production meetings. I seemed to take on the role of his right hand man and helped him with many contacts in the industry, I even made sure I introduced him to Walter when he came over for a convention, after all Walter was my friend and I really wanted him in Legion with us. The writers of the Brittas Empire had suggested to me that my character Patrick would be brought more into the episodes during the last season of shows but that had not been the case, so I had to make a choice and become more and more committed to the Legion project at the expense of my role on Brittas, which in the end turned out to be the wrong choice to make.

The Other Side Of Harry

Mums New Home

My mum had been living with my sister and her two girls in Essex (my sister having divorced her husband Greg some time ago) and a chance had come up for Sue to move into a nice rented house in a picturesque village called Long Melford, and for mum to be given an old persons bungalow not far from her. On hearing the news I was so happy that mum would at last be in a place of her own again and this time she would be in a lovely safe area, to top it all she would also have her own little garden. She used to love the garden in our house in Plaxtol, the only real garden she had ever known, this new house and garden was not in her beloved Kent but after the life she had led in those top couple of rooms at the Elephant, this seemed like Paradise. Mum had stored her few bits of furniture at my sisters, all she had brought from Oswin Street was her dining table, sideboard and two wardrobes, all her pots and pans came too but they were all at least thirty years old. Because the flat I was renting with Carol was too small mum had also looked after a couple of my Star Trek things which I had not sold, and also lots of photo albums and memento's from our past, all our treasured things, nothing worth any money but priceless all the same.

When my mum finally moved into her little bungalow it looked lovely, she was a very clean little lady and housework had been a way of life for her (and sometimes a living) and you could see

287

that she was filled with pride in her new little home, the first time she could actually invite Carol and I around for tea. But as it always seemed to be with my mum's life, fate had a nasty shock in store. Not long after she moved in she had a nasty cold which really brought her down, so she spent a couple of days at my sisters, when she was feeling better she went back to her little bungalow and to her horror she saw that the large water tank in her loft had somehow come crashing down through her ceiling into her bedroom, destroying her bed and all the things around it along with flooding the rest of her home. Among the many things which were destroyed were all of my old Star Trek collectables and so many of our Oswin Street memento's. What the tank missed the water finished off, so many irreplaceable things and memories gone, but not only the things from mums past. The water in the living room had destroyed much of the few bits she had managed to gather for her new home. The only Godsend was that she was not at home when it happened; she would have been killed had she not been at my sisters.

Mum again moved in with Sue while the rebuilding took place, the renovation took a long time but drying out the whole house took very much longer. All of this had an emotional effect on my poor old mum as you could expect, just when her life seemed to be finding some peace at last, fate throws all of this at her again. With no money to speak of we all pulled together to help mum and with the spirit she had always shown, she bounced back saying how lucky she was.

Friend Or Foe

The relationship between Carol and I had seemed to be strange lately, we had been through highs and lows what with trying to get Legion off the ground and then the problems with my poor mum, but we had survived troubled times before and had never argued the way we now seemed to be doing. I put it all down to the fact that we were both in the entertainment industry and were both driven by this will to succeed, the danger of two actors living together is that when one of us would come home rather than saying hello I love you we would often say, has my agent called as our first greeting. I had noticed some other changes too. When I taught in the evenings, mainly Wednesdays our friend Barry the producer would often call and take Carol out for something to eat, he was a friend (or so I thought) so why worry?

Barry professed to be well educated and spoke with a slightly upper class twang, Carol also had a lovely upper class accent and loved the finer things in life and at times I had seemed to sense something between them, but I had dismissed it as my being paranoid. One night Carol was lying in the bath and as I walked in she looked over at me and quite calmly said, I don't love you anymore and I am moving out. I really thought she was joking for a moment but I looked into her eyes and saw that she wasn't, she said that we had grown apart and was telling me this because she would be gone in a week. I felt sick inside as all lovers must do on hearing those words, as Lynne must have done a couple of years before when I left her. I had always felt so guilty about Lynne and had wished so many times, if only I could have turned the clock back. Now it was my turn, what goes around comes around.

With everything happening so fast I had to think about the practical side as well as the emotional side, if Carol left now how could I afford to pay for the flat alone? Then I remembered talking to my friend Tom, he had told me that he was not happy living with his parents but could not afford to get a flat on his own. I called Tom and told him about Carol and I, and at the same time offered him to move in with me and be my flatmate. I had always got on well with Tom and he had been around our flat for dinner many times so I hoped he would jump at the chance and solve both our problems, thank goodness he did. By the end of the week Carol was packed and ready to go, and to be honest the day she left for the last time I was the one with tears streaming down my face, she never batted an eyelid. Much later I found out that when she left me she moved right in to Barry's house, whether it was as a flatmate or something more I never found out, but all I will say is that in the coming months Barry proved to be an expert liar because he never let on where Carol was and played the part of the supportive friend to the hilt (the bastard).

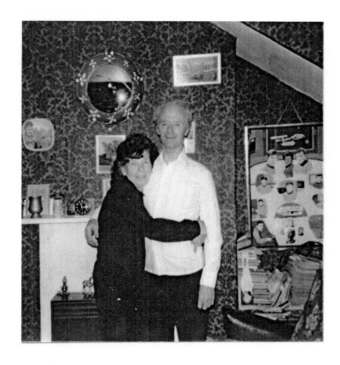

The love that never died. Maggie with her Harry
during the couple of years where he seemed to be
free of his dreaded illness at long last, and they
looked toward some happy twilight years.

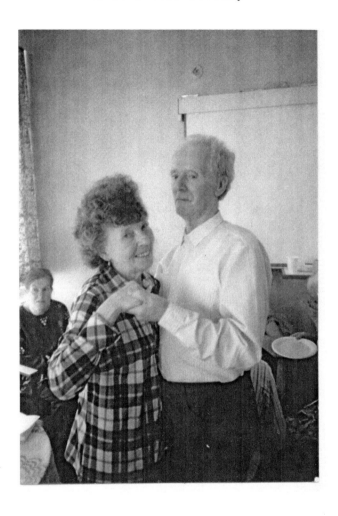

Alas it was not meant to be. Only a couple of years later Alzheimer's again shattered their life. You can see the blank mask which began to take over my fathers face.

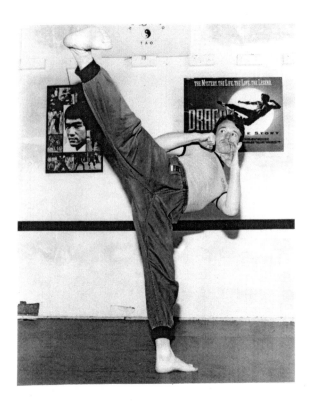

The frightened little John was gone; I had recreated myself out of necessity just to survive.

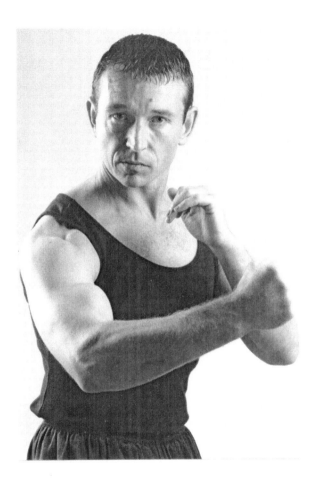

Many people have said to me, it's alright for you, you are a martial arts expert and actor, but what about me I have had it hard. If only they knew.

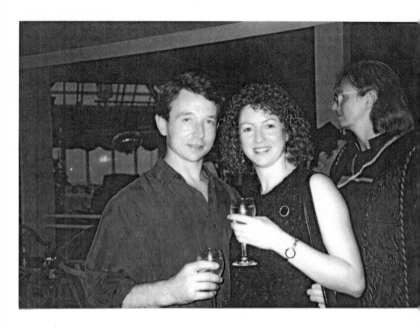

The one, Anne (my Annie) the girl who would
become my future wife and partner for life

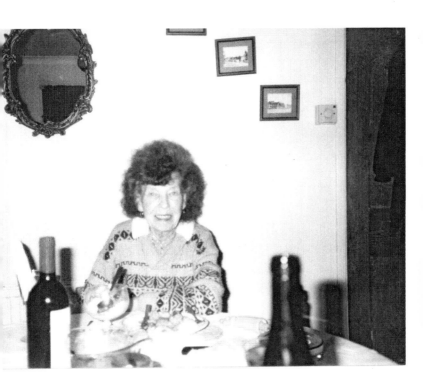

My hero, my mum. The way she will always be in our hearts, smiling and always watching over us.

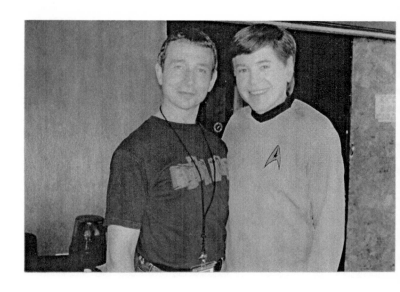

My friend and one of my childhood heroes, Walter
Koenig (Star Treks Mr Chekov) with me on the set
of Star Trek New Voyages.

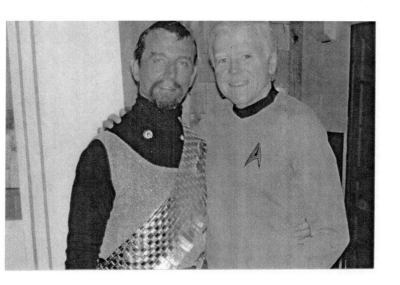

Walter and me. This time I am dressed as Klingon Captain Kargh, and Walter has some fantastic aging make up on. I could never have dreamed all those years ago that I would become part of Star Trek. I just wish mum and dad could have been with me so I could say thank you (yes to Harry too). I know they would have been proud.

The One

Carol moved out and Tom moved in a few days later, I was in a lot of pain over losing her and that pain was mixed in with a great deal of anger too. I had loved Carol and given up a home and a fiancé to be with her and now it all seemed for nothing. But Tom was a good friend and we settled in well together, watching episodes of Friends and eating loads of ice cream to get us through those long womanless nights. Although I did not know it at the time another of my life changing moments was about to occur.

I received a phone call from a place called Pages Bar, it was a Star Trek theme bar in London and I had given a guest talk there earlier in the year, I had also been back there a couple of times for a drink with Carol because it seemed like a fun place (especially for a Star Trek fan). It seemed that Pages had become a focal point for all Star Trek and sci-fi related goings on, including product launches, promotions and TV specials. Bob Benton the manager of the bar told me that Sky were doing a Trek related programme and were going to film it in the bar, they had asked if I would come along and be interviewed on the show and what's more I would be paid a fee. It was just what I needed to get me out of feeling sorry for myself, so I said yes right away. When the interview day came I collected some of my prop collection for them to include in the show and together my flatmate Tom and I boldly went.

When we arrived at the bar the film crew were already set up along with the shows presenter. They had asked for a few Star Trek fans to come along during the day in costume to make the background look more interesting and Trek like, and when the time came for my interview a few fans were asked to sit at tables in the background behind me.   Just before the cameras rolled I turned to say hello to the people in costume who I had never met before, I wanted to thank them for helping out with my interview.   The first person I noticed was this really pretty girl smiling at me, she was dressed in a really great Star Trek Deep Space Nine costume with a figure to match, I actually did a double take when I first saw her. The interview went well and soon it was time for me to go, I sneaked one more look at the pretty lady and headed home.

A couple of weeks went by and I had a call inviting me back to Pages to see the show we had filmed on a big screen in the bar, it was December by now and I was feeling as cold and dark as the nights that were drawing on. I suppose I was still feeling the loss of my father and the more recent loss of my girlfriend although not in so drastic a way, so I thought what a great chance it would be for a night out and I suppose it would also be a bit like the song from the Cheers TV programme (a place where everybody knows my name). Apart from a couple of times in Pages I didn't really ever go to pubs. Being the son of Harry I hardly ever drank and apart from that it would have gone against all the training I did. I also had a real loathing of smoking which led me on a campaign to get my mum out of that terrible addiction (she had smoked since she was fourteen). After years of trying I had finally succeeded and she had not smoked for several years. When I arrived at Pages Bar it was packed and I could see many people in Star Trek uniform. About a third of the people there had taken this night as a chance to swap their business suits and become a starship captain or an alien of some kind which reminded me of when I was a boy and my mum and I would escape all the stress of Harry for a weekend at our beloved conventions, and for a while I too could become Captain Kirk. There were a few off the wall people but on the whole the Trek fans were a bit like football fans wearing their favourite teams colours, and instead of Chelsea it was team Trek.

Bob Benton, the manager, made a few announcements and then we all turned to the big screen to see how the show turned out. I must say that the show looked good and my spot came across well, they also showed a close up of the pretty lady who I had thought about more than once since the show. As the night progressed I signed some autographs (sounds posey I know) and watched all the people having a great time but mainly I stood alone, I was in a strange position, on the one hand like all of the people there I was a Star Trek fan, but on the other I was a professional actor who was involved in Trek from the other side of the fence. I really was that lonely in a crowd person, I guess that was the way I had always felt to a degree because of my unique upbringing, but this time it was for reasons of my own making.

As I stood lost in my actors isolation I felt a hand on my shoulder, it was her, the girl I had seen during my interview shoot, she was standing there smiling at me. She said I hope you don't mind but you look a bit cut off and lonely in the crowd so I thought I would come over for a chat, I told her that she was very perceptive and I did feel a bit that way. She introduced herself as Anne and then apologised saying that she had not realised I was an actor when we had filmed the TV show, she had thought I was just another fan being interviewed but her friends had later told her all the films and TV shows I had been in. She quickly added but I won't treat you any differently just because you are an actor, then she gave me a terrific smile that seemed to go right through me. I learnt that Anne was a legal secretary who worked for a major London law firm, she loved Star Trek and used to be a seamstress, hence the great home made Star Trek uniforms her and her group of friends were wearing. She asked if I would like to join them on their table, but I said no thank you not tonight, she said ok and left me to go back to her friends. I really wanted to join her because I thought she was lovely but I knew I was not ready, my mind was still confused and my heart was still hurt over Carol. I did not talk to her for the rest of the night but I stole a glance at her every so often, she was lovely.

A Christmas Gift

By now Christmas was nearly upon us so everything regarding the film went on the back burner until the New Year and I prepared for my first Christmas in many years without a partner to share it with. This was also Toms first Christmas as my flatmate and I saw it as my chance to let my mum come over to our flat for a pre Christmas visit. For some reason Carol had seemed to resent the strong bond between my mother and I and the fact that since my father passed away we used to speak every day on the phone. Now mum was living near my sister I was not so worried about her but she was still incredibly special to me so this was a great chance to spoil her a little bit and at last cook dinner for her in my own little rented flat. We had a lovely time and by the time her visit was over the snow had begun to fall; it was beginning to look a lot like Christmas.

I had mixed feelings about this holiday season, I had never had loads of friends, I did have lots of students who were sort of removed friends, but the sifu (teacher) barrier had to be and would always be there, apart from Tom my only real friends were in Kent now so I did not know quite what to do about this particular Christmas. Out of the blue as I sat and pondered the festive season to come I had a call from a guy who worked behind the bar in Pages the sci-fi pub. I hardly knew him but he said he had been asked to invite me to a Boxing Day get together by one of the guys from the bar. I nearly said no thanks but then I thought that if I keep saying no thanks to people I could be in for a rather lonely life and I had had enough of that in my younger days. I had said no to the pretty girl in the bar about joining her and her friends for a drink and had regretted it ever since so I said I would meet up with him and we could travel together.

After a train journey across London I met up with the chap from Pages (Chris) and we eventually arrived at a flat in Kings Cross, with me not really knowing why I had been invited to a place I did not know by people I hardly knew. I began to wonder if I had been invited as a token micro celebrity or something. When I walked into the living room I saw that there were people sitting in a circle on the floor playing some kind of card game and as I looked around the circle saying hello to them all I saw her, there she was again looking up at me smiling, the pretty girl named Anne from Pages Bar, it turned out to be a set up. She had told people she had liked me and so without her knowing her friends had arranged all this to get us together. At first Anne went bright red when she saw me and when someone (conveniently) said here John there is a place beside Anne, I think we were both the colour of beetroots. Without saying it we both felt the same attraction, the Christmas I dreaded turned out to be magic, because although I did not know it at the time I had just met the girl who would become my wife, my Annie.

Never Say No To A Klingon

During Christmas and early New Year I saw as much of Anne as I could I even went home to meet her parents in Bedfordshire. I was still doing lots of conventions and work related to Star Trek including being asked to take a team to Birmingham to open the Star Trek exhibition. I had already helped in setting up some aspects of the show and had travelled with it to many cities in the UK to perform and also to help audition people to work at the events. One of the largest portions of the Birmingham exhibition I was asked to put together was a Star Trek quiz, where the prize was a trip to Hollywood and a visit to the Trek sets at Paramount studios. I was also asked to film a load of links for a TV station in full Klingon battle armour from the bridge of the classic Starship Enterprise which was on display. All this was due to go on over Valentines Day as a kind of Valentines Day tie-in, I saw this as my chance.

I had told Anne (who I now called Annie) that I wanted her as part of the cast for the shows at the exhibition because she looked fantastic in her Bajoran Star Trek Deep Space Nine uniform (the one she had been wearing the first time I ever saw her) she agreed to come down with me and the rest of the cast and luck would have it that it fell on a weekend. We all got involved in the quiz show and it ended up with a lovely family winning the trip to Hollywood. I then had to film all of my Klingon TV spots on the bridge in full Klingon battle dress. I had arranged with everyone but Anne that when I said "clear the bridge" they would all go, so as the end of the day drew close I gave the secret (clear the bridge) signal and as if by magic the bridge became empty, I told Annie to hold on for a moment because the press wanted to get a last couple of photographs of her in Captain Kirks chair (a Klingon lie) she obediently sat down in the chair and waited for the press to turn up (which they never did), instead I strode up beside her still in full Klingon battle armour, produced a small box from my Klingon ammunition pouch and put it on the arm of the chair. Annie looked at the box then slowly opened it to reveal a lovely sparkling ring inside; keeping in my Klingon persona I just looked at her and said, "Well!" My lovely Annie looked up at me with a smile and said, "You haven't asked me yet", I melted and became me again saying "Annie will you marry me"? She looked through my Klingon make up and into my eyes and with that incredible smile said "yes". The bridge suddenly exploded with all the people who had been hiding somewhere waiting for the moment, among them was my flatmate Tom and Bob Benton the manager of Pages Bar where we had first met. I was one happy Klingon and that night the champagne flowed.

Legionnaires Disease

Six months had gone since Carol had left and I had heard nothing from Barry or Legion so I decided to call him and arrange a meeting. After speaking to his office a few times Barry finally turned up at my flat. As he walked in the first thing he said was "if you hit me I will have you arrested" which I thought was a strange and stupid thing to say. He then went on to say that he had been worried that I might have somehow blamed him for Carol leaving me, (was it guilt talking?) I told him I thought he was being stupid and that whatever reason had made her leave did not matter; we had a film to produce. With that he calmed down and began to tell me his plans, (but by now he had well and truly planted the seeds of doubt in my mind over him and Carol). Barry told me he had decided to scrap the idea of a series and instead turn it into a movie called "Legionnaires" but he told me that he was having trouble getting backing for the film but he thought he might have come up with a solution. During the past few years a couple of films had been produced using money from a public share issue, which meant that members of the public had paid to become share holders in a film company and in return had been allowed to be extras in the film and receive a percentage from the films profits at the box office, did I think we could do that with our science fiction film? I thought about it for a while and then said a resounding yes.

As a young Star Trek fan I had been to a great many sci-fi conventions and in later years I had moved on to become a guest at those very same conventions, and over the years during my stage shows I had seen how people had loved to hear the story of how I began as one of them in the audience and ended up becoming an actor and mixing on film sets with many of my screen heroes, I also told Barry that through my connections I had access to every sci-fi fan club and convention in the country, I was well known and trusted by the fan community and convention organisers and I felt that by giving people the chance to invest and be in a film alongside their heroes, they would be able to share in some of the fantastic feelings I had treasured when I walked on my first film set. Maybe in this way we could also give some disabled people who I often saw at conventions a chance to be involved in a way they never could have before. It seemed like a great way to get our movie made and help a load of people to make some money and fulfil their dreams at the same time.

Barry and his business partner went into action and after putting all of the legal requirements in place had hundreds of large science fiction posters printed up with the Legionnaires space ship on one side and the share issue prospectus on the other. Included in the prospectus were pictures of all of the leading cast members and when I saw the first copy roll off at the printers I felt a glow of pride, because there I was among those famous faces included in the main cast. The first thing I did was to give a copy to my mum and tell her that she was still my biggest reason to succeed; it would always be for her and for the memory of Harry. The Legionnaires public share issue was all set to go live and my supposed director friend Barry came to see me with all of the plans, I was to be one of the main spearheads of the publicity drive. I had lined up appearances at many conventions and memorabilia shows during the coming year to promote the publicly funded movie and I would be the one on stage talking about Legionnaires due to my high profile in the sci-fi community, it really did seem like a fantastic project and my chance to star in a mainstream big screen movie.

Anne was the sensible one with (as they say) the proper job. I was still teaching the martial arts and had now taken the step up in my acting career to accepting only full dialogue parts in films and TV rather than doing the odd walk on job as well, but time for acting roles became less and less as I become more and more committed to the Legionnaires project, spending as many as three days per week at Elstree film studios doing unpaid pre-production work on the film. I also spent a great deal of time travelling around the country to promote the public share issue so we could raise the funds to actually make the movie, I was the recognisable public face of Legionnaires. I continued to do TV spots and convention talks about why people should support a British sci-fi movie by becoming shareholders and investing in the project, I also put across what a great time they would have appearing alongside us in the film. I was one of the first people to invest £333.00 (the price for a share) and my lovely Annie and her mum Pam also bought their shares, so we really did believe in the project and put our money where our mouth was, so to speak.

It was hard slow going but the money began to come in and after what seemed an eternity the money raised reached a fantastic sum in excess of £860,000. When the share issue had reached that point my friend the producer/director/writer of the film Barry held a little dinner party for all the members of our small team including my now fiancé Annie who had pitched in many times and for long hours to help out. Barry told me in front of everyone that I had been the single driving force behind the whole project even from the days when it was Neil Jackson's Legion, this made me feel great and I really thought we were an unbreakable team.

The next week I was working in the studio putting labels on envelopes to be sent out to prospective shareholders when Barry came over to me and for want of a better word began to bait me into an argument, Barry said, "with all of your martial arts skills and with all of the people who bow to you in your Kung Fu schools, you would still do anything I told you to do just to be in this film, even wear a poxy dress if I asked you, wouldn't you?". I tried to laugh it off but he continued with his insults, he even went as far as to say that it took no intelligence to become an actor or a martial arts instructor and he knew his intellect made me feel threatened. Well I had had enough so I stopped him and replied, "Barry in here you are the director and the boss but outside that all ends and we are equals". I went on to add that I had earned my place in the film many times over without being asked to wear a poxy dress, and that there is a point I would not go beyond even to be in this film. So what was he getting at? We exchanged stares for a moment followed by an awkward silence, then he laughed and patted me on the shoulder and we continued our work. As I have said before I fitted the studio work in whenever I could, usually two or three days per week, but after our conversation days went by without Barry or anyone contacting me.

I decided to call the studio office but every time I did I was told Barry was unavailable. Soon none of my calls were being returned and days turned into weeks, I was never asked back into the studio and I had somehow gone from being Barry's right hand man to being cold shouldered by the whole production team overnight. In my opinion this had been his way of setting me up to argue with him just so he could get rid of me for reasons I can only guess at, but suffice to say that eventually the DTI (the department of trade and industry) were called in and the Legionnaires production was closed down but it was too late. Only a fraction of the shareholders money was left and the film was never made. To cap it all off I later found out that when my ex Carol had suddenly left me it was Barry who behind my back had helped her move out and into his flat....What a great friend and human being that guy turned out to be.

Roots

I was convinced I had at last met my soul mate in Annie and I was finally ready to (as they say) settle down, I also knew just where I wanted to set some roots and live, it was in Kent and as near to Plaxtol as possible. My lovely new fiancé had spent some time with me in Kent and she agreed that was where we should look for our home. I got on well with Anne's mum Pam and my mum was so happy that I had finally met a girl like "me Annie" (as mum would call her) Anne's parents were no longer married but when we all got together for dinner for the first time Stan (Anne's dad) did seem to like me although I did wonder for a moment when he said, remember you make your bed you lie in it? As I later got to know Stan I came to realise that was as close as he was going to come to saying I am glad you are going to marry my daughter, it was just the way he was. He had a face as miserable as sin but it hid a heart as big as a house.

The next year flew by with Annie and me spending as much time together as possible which was not easy, what with my being in Wimbledon and her living with her mum near Luton in Bedfordshire. That made our house hunting in Kent seem all the more urgent, but after viewing only a handful of properties we knew we had found our home. The house we fell in love with was a semi detached perched on a hill overlooking Tonbridge only a few miles from Plaxtol. To this boy from the Elephant and Castle the house on the hill with the apple tree in the front garden seemed like a palace, one of my first thoughts was, mum will love this and I knew dad would have too. When my lovely mum finally got to see our new house tears of joy rolled down her face and it really felt like we had at last come home.

Wedding Bells

Anne Hope became Mrs Anne Carrigan only 18 months after we had first met, we were married in a lovely traditional church in her home village of Barton Le Clay on a beautiful sunny day in May, it really was a kind of fairytale wedding, our wedding cake had Star Trek badges all around the outside and two figures of Captain Kirk and Major Kira (our Trek heroes) standing on the top. It was also a fantastic surprise when Richard Arnold who used to be the assistant to Gene Roddenberry turned up at our wedding. Annie had secretly known he was flying from Los Angeles as a surprise for me. So many of Anne's family had also flown in from Canada and New Zealand for our big day. The only family I had were my mum, sister, my two nieces and little Nathan (my niece Victoria's son, more about Nathan later). If only my dad had still been with us, after all it was him who had created the fire in which I had eventually forged myself into the person I had become and on that special day as I looked around me it seemed that finally the son of Harry had done ok.

But if my father had lit the fire it was my incredible mother who had always been there to pull me from the flames before they consumed me, and as well as my lovely new wife, in my heart that day was for her too, top of the world ma. After our wonderful ceremony we began our evening celebrations and I had the first dance with my lovely Annie, we danced to our song, a "perfect year" by Dina Carol, then to Annie's song by John Denver which I had always loved. The next dance had to be with my mum who had found no reason to dance for many years, as we danced I looked into her smile and at last I saw her happy.

Our wedding nearly did not happen though all because of me, Mr Bullet proof John. Only a few weeks before the wedding I had been teaching a stocky Police officer from London and we were doing some light boxing (joke) I had caught him with a couple of punches and I think frustration set in. All of a sudden he let loose a massive right cross which caught me square in the left eye. Now he was wearing big old 18 ounce gloves but even with those on I knew I had a problem. As I staggered back from the punch and stopped for a moment it really was like something out of a cartoon. I looked up and I could see three of everything through my left eye. We stopped for a while and he was full of apologies, no way was that punch from a light spar. It took about ten minutes for my eye to get back to normal before we could carry on but I felt ok. When the lesson finished I had a follow on lesson right after, I had a headache (who wouldn't) but I was otherwise ok. I started the lesson and was showing how to punch and get power by blowing out through your nose as you strike. I punched and blew, then looked up to see the horrified look on my students face. I turned to the mirror to see that the left side of my face under my eye had blown up and was literally hanging off like some massive water balloon. No air had come out of my nose it had somehow all gone into my eye socket. I was rushed off to hospital for x-rays and it was found that I had a fractured eye socket; they said that I needed to see a specialist in London who dealt with these problems. When I got home to Annie and she saw my face she actually started to heave, she was mortified; our wedding was only two weeks away.

I went to the specialist in London who told me that they might have to give me surgery to repair the fracture but also that the surgery could leave me with a slight speech impediment because they would have to go up through the roof of my mouth, an actor with a speech impediment, oh no. He asked me how it had happened and I told him I was a martial artist and also told him about my imminent wedding. He surprised me by saying he did the martial arts too. He then said I am going to give you two weeks to try and heal yourself, I believe we martial artists can tap into healing properties that other people often can't. He said that I had two weeks to evacuate the air from my eye otherwise they would have to go in through my mouth to repair my eye. I went home and focused somehow on the eye repairing and the air coming out. Thank God somehow it did, and the wedding and my acting career was saved, but I was told that I could not risk anymore damage to that eye, I had been lucky.

After that incident Annie banned me from sparring without a head guard and I agreed, any more hits to that eye and my sight could be permanently damaged but just a few months after our wedding I had another problem.

Challenges

I had had quite a few martial arts challenges throughout the years, mainly when I was much younger and they had all been silly ego based ones which I had coped with (and won) without doing anyone any permanent damage. I now saw that kind of thing as stupid and was against all I believed in about the martial arts but....One day I was in my club after a long day teaching when a guy walked in, he was bald with tattoos and was extremely well built. I recognised him from paying a visit to my club and joining in with a lesson a couple of weeks before. I walked over to say hello but I could tell by the look on his face we had a problem. He said that the martial arts school where he trained was founded by an instructor who had issued a challenge to Bruce Lee but Bruce had refused to fight (as if), that instructor had now (like Bruce) passed on so it was up to us to settle this score with me being a third generation Bruce Lee student, he also said he was a European kick boxing champion. I said that I no longer did the stupid challenge thing especially not for so worthless a reason; I said that he had nothing to prove to me. With that he spit in my face, because I had made sure I kept my distance from him I missed most of it but that was enough.

I told him that I did not want to cause a problem where I worked (my school was in a fitness centre in a golf club) so we agreed to go across into a nearby field. We walked in silence and I could hardly believe this was happening, I had not long got over the injury to my eye and I promised Annie I would no longer take any silly risks. I wanted to turn and say look we have to call this off, but my pride would not let me, also somewhere deep inside a part of me was doing this for Bruce (stupid I know).

When we got to the field he pulled on a little pair of leather driving gloves and that was it this was for real. No boxing gloves and no protection. My mind and heart were racing and my mouth was dry, what if he got my injured eye, what if...then a calmness came to me and my training kicked in. We nodded as a slight sign of respect and he was on me. This guy attacked me as if he hated me, he was big, fast, skilled and committed. I did what my years of training had taught me to do and boy did I need it all. I was not at my best, it had been a long day I was tired, and to be honest I was preoccupied with not getting my eye damaged. I absorbed a lot of blows mainly from his legs, and he took all I could throw at him too. His heart was all in this fight while I did not really want to be there, it had been forced upon me.

It turned out that we fought tooth and nail for fifteen minutes until I had almost had enough. The big mad bald guy shouted a tirade of obscenities as he tried a big front kick. I remember blocking it with the bottom of my right foot and shouting myself as I waded in throwing continuous straight punches to his face, one two and three hit and I followed up with a sickening elbow across his temple, he went down with blood filling the air behind him. I stood in shock, I thought he was dead. I quickly bent down to check on his breathing and for a few moments he did not move. I could hardly see his face for the blood which seemed to come from everywhere. All of a sudden he moaned and began to stir (thank God) He grabbed his t-shirt and stuffed it in the wounds on his face as I helped him up. I said we should go to a hospital but he just shrugged me off, turned to me, bowed and said, "you're the hardest C...I have ever fought".   Then he staggered off. I have no idea where he went. By the time I got home my body had all but seized up. I walked through the door to find Annie waiting for me. Right away she said, what's wrong. I had hardly a mark on my face because I had protected my eye so well but I could not hide, the rest of my body and legs had been through a war. I let my trousers fall to the floor and from the top to the bottom. My left leg was a mass of congealed blood under the skin which had pooled to the lower part of my leg turning it a mass of black. Annie went mad.

I am not proud of what happened that day and the sheer sickening violence of it all nearly turned me off of my beloved martial arts. I had been forced to do that to another human being not as a last resort to protect myself or my family but simply through ego or some other worthless emotion, could I (should I) have walked away that day and lost face, yes I should. What if one of us had died, for what?

The Siege

My niece Victoria had fallen pregnant a couple of years ago when she was only fifteen and I remember being really shocked and disappointed at the time but as they say, these things happen. Victoria's boyfriend had all kinds of problems and the two of them warred frequently. Torrs (as we called her) had split from him and was living in a council house with her young son Nathan and I had not seen her for some time, although I would always be kept informed by my sister about the on going situation. One day I received a call from Torrs herself and she said that she had been threatened by Nathan's father who told her he would be coming to take her son away, and since that call he and some of his cronies had almost laid siege to the house. Well, Victoria was my niece and she had turned to me, how could I not be there for her.

My sister arranged for Victoria and Nathan to secretly leave the house while I had travelled down and just as secretly slipped in, the police had been called several times over this issue but after a while I think it became like the boy who cried wolf to them so they could not be counted on all the time. With Victoria and little Nathan safely out of the way I waited inside the house with Sue. There were a few callers during my first few hours in the house, some were Victoria's friends and some were from the gang of creeps who were never far away. I stayed hidden while my sister had told the latter uninvited visitors to piss off which they did, mouthing veiled threats as they went, they must have thought they were terminators because one turned around and dramatically said I'll be back. I was not sure just what I was supposed to do but in my mind I thought eventually they would try to break into the house looking for Nathan or to try and do damage to Victoria or the house, so with all of my years of training I was going to be ready to teach them a lesson. I had heard that some of these creeps were on drugs and I knew what drugs did to people, so I was under no illusions as to what I could be up against, but I was ready and determined to protect my family.

As night time fell at the end of the first day I rigged all the doors and windows with trip wire and placed martial arts weapons at different points all over the house (if anyone came in armed I would be too). I waited up all night downstairs while my sister got some sleep upstairs, the situation seemed unreal but it felt a lot like the feelings I had during my time as a bodyguard, only this time it was personal. The long night passed without incident but with a few false alarms, the next day found the return of Nathan's father and some of his friend's one of whom was a martial artist. I had given a demonstration to him during more friendly times and shall we say I dented his ego a bit. This visit saw the lads full of themselves and giving their views to my sister who they thought was all alone, as they were in mid tirade I stepped into view in the doorway and just looked at them with a slight smile on my face, they all knew who I was and for some reason they did not look happy, I wonder why? They requested that they be allowed into the house to get something which Nathan's dad had left in the loft, we agreed to let one of them come in to retrieve whatever it was. As he climbed the ladder to the roof I watched him closely and surprised him by saying, "oh by the way if you go anywhere near that knife hidden under your shirt you had better know how to use it". I lightened the situation by adding, "but you might need it, the spiders are really big in the loft". Needless to say the knife stayed tucked away. In the end no violence or force was used thank God and Nathan ended up in the best place for him at the time living with a woman who had rescued another small boy long ago, with care sacrifice and love, her name was Maggie Carrigan.

New Starts And New Nanny

It was a time for new beginnings, I was in my lovely new home with my lovely new wife, a married man at last (I had escaped long enough) and my mum was living in a little bungalow with her own little garden, a lovely little boy to again look after and my sister just around the corner. My niece Victoria was not a bad mother but she had lived with turmoil and drama's of one kind or another for some time and she was just not ready or able to give Nathan the time and care he needed, so he had moved in with my mum who doted on him and saw it as her chance to look after him and give him the love she had given me when I had so needed it most. As always the amazing thing, was that she was going to do it all again while still having next to nothing herself, although this time around she was not alone.

Nathan grew into a lovely well mannered little boy during the time he spent with mum and in the early days he called her 'new nanny' which always made me smile. My life with Annie got off to a stormy start unfortunately with the two of us having many head to head rows during our first year, we loved each other but we were both strong characters and Anne had never lived away from home before. She had lived alone with her mother for some years and the two of them had learned to make the decisions and survive very well together, two strong woman against the world sort of thing, while I had lived away from home in quite a few different situations throughout the years and as the strong willed martial artist and actor I too had become used to being the master of my own destiny, hence the clash. As time went on we learned to compromise and join forces with our wills and rather than butting heads we became a good team.

Patience My Arse

I was married, happy, finally back in my beloved Kent and my martial arts teaching was going well…but still it burned inside me, the wish, no the need to make something of myself in the film or TV industry but nothing was happening. The Brittas Empire had ended, the Legionnaires movie came to nothing and the last real role I played had been a couple of years earlier when I had been on stage at the Hackney Empire portraying the actor David Garrick for the factual TV series called Connections.

Being a follower of Bruce Lee's teachings I was aware of just what a fantastic self motivated person he was, and something about him sprang to mind. He was also an actor as well as the worlds best martial artist and when he felt his life had slowed and he was in a rut with no work coming in he would hang a poster on the wall behind his desk, on the poster were two vultures sitting on a cactus in the middle of the desert, they were looking down at a pile of bones and one vulture was saying to the other, "patience my arse, I'm going to kill something". Which was all about not being like a vulture who has to wait for something to fall down and die before it can eat, metaphorically you have to go out and kill something, get what you want and don't just wait and hope, so I made up my mind to do something which very few people (if any) had done before.

I sat and wrote a shooting script for a training video which I called 'Need To Know Self Defence', it would be a self defence instructional tape aimed at ordinary men and women, such as office workers who have to work late at night, doctors, nurses, anyone who had ever felt the hair standing up on the back of their neck as they walked a dark street. I spent a long time in deciding just what should be in the tape and I tested all of the woman's moves out with Annie to make sure a woman could do them effectively, I then went to a couple of my private students who I thought might be interested in financing the project. I raised seven thousand pounds and then took out a loan for another thousand myself to add to it. So with my shareholders in place I now needed a female co presenter to present the woman's portion along with me, a director, a studio and a crew. I had produced my own film before (The Need) and had many friends in the industry so before too long a director, studio and crew were all in place which just left a co presenter. I contacted an actress named Jill Greenacres who I had worked with on The Brittas Empire, we got on well and I knew she had done some kind of martial arts training, when I met Jill and explained what I had in mind she was eager to get involved and I thought she would be perfect for the part. As time for the shoot grew closer we rehearsed as much as possible, I had some of my students acting as thugs and attackers in the video so I had time to prepare them all but time was limited with Jill.

On the day before the shoot I was going through a last minute rehearsal with her when she misjudged an elbow technique and POW, her elbow hit me just above my top lip. I managed to role with the blow but it was too late and blood rolled down my face. When I got to the mirror my heart sank, I had a wide gash above my lip which I knew would need stitches, Jill was mortified and she and her boyfriend Richard rushed me to casualty. As I sat waiting to be seen I could feel the swelling above my mouth getting bigger. I had booked and paid for the studio along with accommodation for the cast and crew and we were due to start filming at seven am the next day, how? I would look a mess, would I even be able to talk, let alone the pain I knew I would be in, how could we do it? It was the arrow and the rock all over again. To cut a long story short, I explained the situation to the doctor in the hospital so he agreed to give me butterfly stitches instead of thread which would be easier to cover with makeup (I hoped) he also gave me load of pain killers. I had no sleep that night but there we all were next morning ready to go, the old saying is true (the show must go on). I put a thin base make up all over my face to try and hide the three plaster stitches and we shot all of my scenes in an extra low moody light, as I turned during the shots you could see the stitches if you knew they were there and from a side view my top lip looked like something from planet of the apes. But the hardest part was delivering my lines through the pain and not slurring my words or fluffing my lines.

The cut had gone all the way through my lip to the inside of my mouth and boy did it smart.

The video came out very well and some of my students did a great job as the attackers and defenders both inside the studio and on some outdoor scenes. I used the last of the investor's money to hold a launch party at Pages Bar (where I first met my Annie) and Jill and I invited many family friends and people we knew from the industry, but to me as always the guest of honour was my lovely mum. Early on in this book I wrote about the first movie I was ever involved with called Melody with Jack Wild and Mark Lester, well the world had turned full circle for me when into my launch party walked not only the cast from the Brittas Empire but also a friend of Jill's, Jack Wild who I had so looked up to those long years ago. We swapped memories of Melody and of our youth and for me that really was the icing on the cake. The guests had a good time eating, drinking and watching Need to know Self Defence on a big screen, I just wish that Harry could have been there to see his son; I know he would have been proud. I have to add a sad footnote here because during the writing of this book Jack Wild also sadly passed away, but I am so glad we had the chance to be together on that special night.

If At First You Don't Succeed

After the launch of Need to know Self Defence I spent months sending out sample copies to distributors and TV stations, I also did some newspaper interviews and was even asked to talk about the video and self defence live on a top London radio station, but it was all to no avail. The feedback I received from the distributors was that although they liked the video there was no other one out on the market to compare it with so they were not sure how it would sell, no one was prepared to take a chance on it. I even heard back from one place saying that because the subject was about being attacked they felt normal people might not want to hear about violence (that's right stick your head in the sand). Although all my efforts had again come to nothing the dream of making it in the industry still burned.

As I have said, throughout the years I had been a guest at many Star Trek and media conventions performing my talks, stunt shows and demonstrations, one day I received an offer to be a guest at a big three day event called Gen Con, this was a sort of convention for people who liked role playing games and re enactment societies, it was to be held on a university campus and they were expecting over five thousand people. I had been asked to put on three workshops per day on screen fight choreography for all the various Vikings, Vampires, Hobbits and other assorted weird and wonderful beings attending the convention, all for just a couple of hundred pounds for the whole weekend. I began to have second thoughts because the money offered did not seem much for all the work that would be involved, that was until I looked at the other guests who were invited to the con. Included as part of the guest list were the director, writer and cast of a new proposed science fiction show called First Frontier, the cast included some well known names from sci-fi such as Claudia Christian from a show called Babylon 5 and Jeremy Bulloch who played Boba Fett in Star Wars, this was it, my chance. I turned to Annie and said I will be a guest at this con and by the time I come home I will have a part in this new series. As the saying goes, once the doorway is in sight the pathway is irrelevant.

I booked into the campus and the long weekend began, it was a first for me to be staying in the enclosed world of a college environment surrounded by all manner of weird goings on (and I thought Star Trek conventions could be a little strange). I began the first of my three workshops per day and it turned out great, I was a hit and had people booking in for the next show as the last one finished, and by the second day I heard people talking about that little guy who can really kick ass (I wonder who that could be?) I made it my job to talk to the other guests over the weekend especially the producer writer and cast from First Frontier and I invited them to come and see my last show of the weekend, many of them turned up but unfortunately not the creator/producer. I pulled out all the stops for my last show and chose my moment to ask for a volunteer to help in a demonstration, I looked in the audience and saw a guy from First Frontier saying, you will do nicely. I finished by kicking a bottle off of his head after creating the big build up. I finished to roaring cheers. He came up to me after the show and said, have you got any info about yourself we could have? I said it just so happens that I have and produced my CV photo and video show reel, which is just what I had planned for and the whole reason I had gone to the con in the first place. Two days later I was teaching a lesson when my mobile rang, it was the writer/producer of First Frontier Andrew Dymond, he said that he had just viewed my show reel and thought I was fantastic (I was dumb struck) he then asked if we could meet up in London to talk about my working on the series (wow), I was blown away, my go get it attitude about being seen by the right people at the convention had worked and I arranged to meet Mr Dymond the following week. When Annie came home from work she found me grinning from ear to ear and doing the 'this could be the chance' dance. In short I was ecstatic, all I had ever wanted was the chance to show someone who mattered in the industry what I could do, now a producer writer director had seen and liked what he saw, I phoned mum right away to tell her and as always she said,

I know you are going to make it son, I replied I am mum, for you and for dad.

The following week could not come fast enough and I arrived at Leicester Square to meet Mr Dymond. Andrew arrived with a girl named Sue, who as well as being his assistant turned out to also be his fiancé. Over lunch we seemed to hit it off right away and seemed to have so much in common, apart from our love of the film and TV industry Andrew also loved science fiction and super heroes. I had always loved the Marvel character of the Mighty Thor God of Thunder and Andrew loved Iron Man, another Marvel creation. At the end of our meeting we agreed that somehow we had to work together. In the months that followed I saw a lot of Andrew, both professionally and socially with each of us visiting the others homes, Anne and I also attended some pre-publicity launches for First Frontier where I was introduced as the newest member of the cast and it felt good. After all we had been through with Legionnaires I really wanted Annie to be proud of me by my finally making it into a series or film again, but...it was not meant to be.

The finance for the series collapsed and it was shelved, it seemed I was destined to have my dreams snatched away at the last minute yet again. My friendship with Andrew remained though and he continued to say that he really thought I had talent and that he would create a starring vehicle for me to showcase it in. Andrew was true to his word and together with a great writer name Jeff Evans and input from me he created a great script for a movie called Download, a light hearted martial arts action thriller, the script was fantastic and we were back on track. It was during this time that Andrew and Sue were due to be married and it came as a great shock when Andrew asked me to be his best man, it was an honour and I agreed right away. We came up with the idea that Andrew, Sue, Annie and I would all go to California together by way of a honeymoon for the two of them, after all that is where the dreams of most people in the industry lie.

The wedding turned out fine and soon it was time for the newlyweds and us to jet off to the land of make believe, Hollywood. I had always felt bad about the crap I had involved my friend Walter Koenig in over the failed Legionnaires so I was still determined to somehow one day work with him. I decided to contacted him about Download and to my joy Walter said that if the script was good and the money could be put in place he would love to play the lead bad guy to my hero in the film, we even hooked up with him in LA during our visit to talk about the project but…you guessed it, soon after our return from the states Andrews friend and fellow script writer Jeff Evans suddenly died, and as if it was not bad enough losing such a nice guy, the Download script was then legally tied up by Jeff's family so it could not be used. Now you see why this chapter is called if at first you don't succeed. Boy keeping positive is not an easy thing to do when fate keeps snatching those dreams out right from under your nose, but the truly sad thing about all of this was the passing of a really nice human being, Jeff.

Once More Unto The Breach

If my life and all my years of training had taught me anything it was that you only fail when you give up trying, so I again swallowed my disappointment and threw myself back into training my body (as always) and honing my acting skills, (when preparation meets opportunity success begins) and I was not going to be caught napping when (not if) the opportunity came (as I had always believed it must). Some time went by and Andrew again came to see me, he had yet another idea (which was his strongest attribute). He wanted to create the worlds first fully interactive science fiction, fantasy, martial arts movie where the viewer could change the outcome of the film by making multiple choices as the story went along, and with today's equipment and DVD technology it would be possible, it was a fantastic idea but would be very hard to do with live actors, that is one of the reasons no one had done it before, so I said great lets go for it.

Andrew spent weeks writing the incredibly complex script with all of its multiple choice pathways but by the time it was finished it was amazing how he had tied it all together, but now how do we film it? There were fifty alternate pathways in the story with dozens of fight scenes, as well as loads of special effects. The story centres around four ordinary somewhat introverted people who get sucked through a vortex from different time periods on Earth and find themselves in a crazy world called Argonia where they find they have become the secret Heroes they have always felt lurked inside themselves. They are forced to fight demons giants, vampires and dragons to name but a few of the bad things they encounter. During a script meeting I had with Andrew I had the chance to help create my character, to really mirror my own life, my character (Marshall) turns from a somewhat timid Star Trek fan into a martial arts expert with muscles (sound familiar) and becomes the hero he had always wanted to be. Now Andrew was going to fund this venture out of his own pocket so I signed on as associate producer on the project as well as fight choreographer, casting director, location scout, prop maker, make up and sfx man, acting and stunt coach, and oh yes a little thing called leading actor (not much to do really). Once more unto the breach dear friends.

Argonia Or Bust

Andrew set dates for us to start filming in the early summer of 2001 and left it to me to suggest people who I thought might be good as the other characters in Advanced Warriors (the title of the film) I had already contacted an actress called Chase Masterson from Star Trek Deep Space Nine, who I had met at a convention and it looked like she would be interested in playing one of the four main roles, Andrew knew an actor from Star Wars named Jeremy Bulloch who was to have been in Andrews other show (First Frontier) and it also looked like Jeremy was on board with us, which left one more main part to cast. I knew a pretty young actress from my Carol days who I had introduced to my (then) best friend Mike, her name was Rebecca Nichols and I thought she would be perfect for the part, the only problem was that the character was supposed to be a great fighter, but Rebecca had only done acting and modelling, she was very fit but had never thrown a punch in her life. One more fairly large role was to be filled by an actor (and producer) who had spent some years as Dr Who's sidekick, his name was Mark Strickson, Star Trek, Star Wars and Dr Who in one film with me as the leading man…this could be fun.

In the film we still had to fill loads of other more minor roles, but it did seem that all of the other characters would also need to have some kind of martial arts or action background. We had three months till we began filming so I put it to Andrew that the other characters in AW had to do far more screen fighting than they had acting and lines, so it seemed logical that it would be easier to give some of my martial arts class acting lessons for the three months than it would be to train actors to fight in so short a time. He agreed and auditions were held in my martial arts school with Andrew and I as the judges. Some of my class had acted in my self defence video and on some stunt shows with me before, I had even got a couple of them on some TV and film projects with me so some were more used to the camera than others. It did not take us long to choose who would be right for the roles and so began the three months of intensive drama, martial arts and stunt training, which included turning Rebecca into a kick ass heroine along with turning all my other people into passable actors as well as stunt fighters. I had to somehow fit all this in with learning my own lines, choreographing over thirty fight scenes, scouting locations and making props. All of these tasks I had stepped up to do were daunting and would consume my every waking (and sometimes sleeping) moment, but my belief system which I had tried hard to cultivate told me I could do it.

As filming drew closer and the pressure grew more intense I began to feel the demons of my past calling to me and I began to be troubled by self doubts. I was to be the leading male actor in this film and I would be working alongside a veteran British actor who had not only been in one of the biggest films in history (Star Wars) but had also been in many TV series as well as three James Bond movies. Then there was Chase Masterson who had come from Hollywood and been in Star Trek as well as many other Hollywood productions during her career, would my acting hold up beside them? Would I be any good, what if I forgot my lines or became tongue tied? These demons had in one form or another haunted me all of my life, whenever I was about to undertake any big thing, like the martial arts tournaments, the stunt team tests, the fight challenges and on and on, those demons of self doubt went way beyond what everyone feels now and again, they were the legacy left to me by the life my family had led with Harry. I had always felt these fears and doubts but had always forced myself to rise above them, to succeed in spite of or because of them, I have never known which. Those self doubts were why I had always thrown myself into things which especially in my early life I was so ill equipped to do, maybe to prove to myself (and to the world) and shout "see I can not only do them I can be the best at them". The boy who was beaten up became the martial arts expert, the boy who found it hard to mix with people after being a virtual prisoner for years became the extrovert actor, on stage in front of hundreds of people or on camera in front of millions. But sometimes it all catches up with me and it takes every effort to tell the doubt demons just what to do with themselves, when that happens I take a deep breath and just get on with following my dreams. I saw Advanced Warriors as my last big chance to make it in the film industry, I still wanted to make it for mum and for the memory of my dad, but now I also had Annie to think of and to make proud of me, I wanted to give her a secure future not just one filled with missed and broken chances.

I had spent many weeks of rehearsal, putting my people and Rebecca through their paces, I also spent hours scouting locations in which to film. The hardest location to find was a large forest we could use which was supposed to be on the planet Argonia. During all my years in Plaxtol I had been fortunate to get to run around in many magic woodlands so I re-visited some of them and eventually found the perfect place, another plus was that it was only a few miles from Tonbridge where I lived. On one of his visits I took Andrew to the forest and he agreed, it looked like Argonia. That was the deciding factor; we would base most of the filming in Kent that summer. We did have one terrible set back though even before a single scene had been filmed, with only a couple of weeks to go before principle photography began the whole of the country became quarantined as the terrible foot and mouth disease ravaged the land, which meant all forests were now no go areas. We had paid for and put in place all the permits needed for filming in a national forest for the two weeks of the shoot, and now that was all to be postponed and re-arranged. I had lost a commercial which would have earned me £3000 because filming it would have it clashed with filming AW (and three grand to me was like three million) so now it turned out I had lost it for nothing.

We eventually began filming a bit later than planned but it was no use crying over spilled milk. We used my home and the home of (Jen) one of my students who was in the film as our unit bases, Jen had a lovely historical ex pub as her home with large grounds and land to go with it and Jen's back garden became part of the enchanted forest of Argonia for the filming. Jen and her husband (Keith) also put up and fed many of the crew who had come down from Bristol, they were a God send. Annie and I put up Andrew and Sue and also held many cast and crew dinners while we all watched the dailies (the film footage which had been shot that day), I must say that my lovely Annie was a brick during filming and would come home after a long day working in London to begin a long night looking after a house full of actors, but she knew I had so much riding on AW and had worked hard for so long to get this far. The filming was really gruelling physically and emotionally and I really do not know how everyone got through it, but we did and as the last shot was filmed I know we all felt we had done our best.

The shooting wrapped with hugs cheers kisses (and a few black eyes from the fight scenes), but we were full of hope for what Advanced Warriors could become. When the rest of the cast and crew had gone home Chase Masterson checked out of her hotel and stayed with Annie and I for a couple of days, which meant two Star Trek cast members had stayed in our guest room (maybe we should put up a blue historical plaque above the bed) Chase was a lovely house guest and was a pleasure to be with, but she did not share our optimism over AW, I hoped she was wrong?

The Launch

Long months of post production followed for the massive amount of special effects needed, and then the build up to the release our double DVD, complete with the making of video, interviews and my own Need to know Self Defence as part of the extras. During those months the cast interviews for the DVD extras were completed and some added footage was shot of scenes which had not quite worked or had been left out because of lack of time. To really give our film a push I thought we needed some kind of media press launch so I took it on myself to organise it, I booked a bar in London which was run by one of my students and sent out invitations to the media and celebrities who I had some kind of contact with, the invites also included all the cast crew and friends of Advanced warriors. I was able to pull all of this together for a fraction of the normal price by using my contacts and asking friends for favours. I felt I had been working towards this night for many years and the only guest I really wanted there was the one person I owed everything to, my mum. After all we had been through together I wanted this night to be for her as a way of finally saying, we made it ma. I found a small hotel in London for my mum and my sister; I wanted them both to share in the feelings of our night. The evening was a great success and as the film's leading man it was up to me to give a speech, I got through it without any Oscar type tears but inside me I held all the memories of what my family had been through to bring us to this night, and I knew that somewhere Harry was looking down smiling with his thumb in the air.

I was given a copy of Advanced Warriors and apart from being critical of my own work (as all actors are) I thought it was great and I was proud of it. We also had our public launch at a big sci-fi convention called The SF Ball, where people could buy AW for the first time, response was fantastic and we all signed autographs together (including Chase and Jeremy), we also did a question and answer session on stage as clips of AW were shown, it was an amazing time and we continued to be guests at many other conventions and shows around the country to promote our epic adventure. We even appeared on a prime time TV chat show, and I got an incredible buzz when I went to a big London sci-fi and comic store and there on the shelves was Advanced warriors, we had made it...or had we? As AW began to sell and some good feedback began to come in we were dealt a crushing blow, some people began to return their copies of the film saying that it just froze on their DVD player during the interactive portions of the film (which was most of it). For some reason certain makes of player coped with it fine and it was great, but others it would just not work on. It turned into a nightmare and no more discs could be sent to shops, the problem would take a lot of time and money to fix and the company had neither. The disc was eventually re-cut into a new version but it was too late the momentum was lost. As of this writing the new AW has been sent to new distributors but as yet no one has picked it up and no one has made any money, in fact it has cost everyone dearly in more than just time. But Andrew being ever the tryer has said that AW will now be released as one of the first interactive movies available on mobile phones sometime in the future. We will have to see.

So, just as the dream seemed to have at last come true, it had yet again crashed at my feet, it felt as if my last chance had gone when I had so believed that one day I would make something of myself in the film world. As always mum was there to bolster me up with don't worry luv it will turn out alright, when one door shuts another one opens, you never know what's hanging till it drops. Well this door did seem well and truly shut and there seemed nothing good left to drop, and so I half heartedly knuckled down to continue teaching and although it really hurt me to do so part of me resigned myself to just being Kung Fu John as, my friend Ron used to call me, maybe my life as an actor was just not meant to be.

Dread

I had piled all my hopes and dreams of any kind of success in the industry onto Advanced Warriors and now it again seemed a million miles away. I had invested over a year of my life into the project and because I was proud of it I had sent copies to all of my friends over in Hollywood saying it would be out in shops world wide very soon, now I felt stupid, they say that pride comes before a fall, boy were they right. I tried to see all the wonderful things I should be grateful for not the things I did not have, as my wonderful mum had always done throughout her life, to be where I was with all that I had should be more than enough for the boy from Oswin Street. Life went on and as always mum would ring me every morning (unless I called her first) but I began to pick up on something in her voice, as if she was just saying things to keep me happy when I would ask how she was, as if she were keeping something inside, I was soon to find out that my suspicions were true.

My mum had always put herself last in life, she would go hungry to feed someone, she had committed herself to looking after my little nephew Nathan with the same kind of unconditional love she had given my sister and I during our dark struggling early years. I found out later that my mum was sleeping on her little sofa in her little living room while Nathan had her bed, she had done this for a couple of years now and I could not believe I had not realised it. Annie and I had made sure that we visited mum and Nathan every few weeks and we tried to see to it that they had the things she could not afford, a good TV, a video, a new vacuum cleaner, kettle and so on. Sue was always on hand to help but she had no money herself so we helped when we could. Mum was looking after Nathan on her pension alone which was hardly anything, but he was a lovely happy well mannered highly intelligent little boy. She had done a fantastic job of giving him the stability he needed, it was like looking at myself all over again when I looked at Nathan, I had had a super mum to rescue me, he had a super Nan to rescue him.

Annie and I had a virtually new single bed just sitting in our garage and when we found out where mum had been sleeping we knew what we had to do. My lifelong friend Mike who had donated the TV to my mum offered to help me take the bed down to her, so we literally strapped it on to the roof of his car and drove the long trek to Suffolk where she lived. As we drew up at the end of our long slow journey mum came out onto her little pathway to meet us as she always did, but for the first time in my life I did not see the neat little lady who no matter what she had been through always had pride in the way she looked, this time I saw that her hair was untidy, she was still clean and lovely but she looked painfully thin and ill, and when she drew closer I could see that somehow a light had gone from her eyes. We had our usual big hug but I could not help saying, mum something's wrong isn't it? She was as always full of bravado and put on one of her famous fronts, but I was really worried, a look between me and Mike told me that he felt the same. We unloaded the bed and you would have thought we had given her the crown jewels, she had cakes and loads of food for us which she would not let us refuse, but this time I made sure that she sat down while I acted as tea boy. We had a lovely day with her but when it was time to leave her I left with a terrible feeling of dread inside me.

The Longest Night

After seeing my mum looking so thin and tired I could not get her out of my mind, she had told me that her loss of weight had been due to her being diagnosed recently with an illness called dumps disease, this illness causes all of your food to pass right through you instead of letting it be stored as fat or goodness in your body, but the doctor had told her they could control it ok. Why had she not told me about it before? I was used to mum keeping things from me to stop me worrying but why this if it was not that serious? I told her we would need to get her built up, maybe with protein drinks, but I still had this feeling of dread deep inside of me. I started to phone my sister more to ask how mum was, because mum always had the stock reply of, I'm fine love, no matter how she felt, then she would add, don't worry about no one or nuffink. Sue said that she was really worried about mum because during a short walk she seemed to almost gasp for breath and had to turn back and go home, this from a woman who even after she turned seventy still used to kick her leg up above her head to show us she was still young. Sue and I started to have daily conversations about mum's condition after that one night I called mum as I always did and this weak little voice answered, I felt a sudden rush of fear, I said mum what's wrong you sound terrible, she replied, I am not well boy I need help. God that was the first time in my life I had ever heard her ask for anything.

I called my sister on her mobile and she was already on her way with my niece Catalina. When Sue saw mum she phoned for an ambulance right away and mum was rushed to hospital, I wanted to go to her but Sue assured me there was no need and she would keep me informed what was going on as soon as possible. I couldn't settle till I finally heard back from Sue, the diagnosis was that mum had a severe chest infection but they were only keeping her in hospital for a day and a night Sue said she wished they would keep her in longer, she was still very worried about mum. When she came home and I finally spoke to her on the phone she was a frail and breathless voice, but still she only thought of my feelings and said, "don't worry boy I signed a contract to live till I get me telegraph from the Queen".

It turned out that Sue had found a temporary job where she could earn some much needed cash but it meant going away for a few days, and as timing would have it it was for the weekend just after mum came home, no way could my mother be left on her own in her condition so I said I would be down to look after her. Annie had a million things to do so she could not stay with me but as long as I was there with me old cockney sparrow looking after her that's all I really cared about. Annie took me down to mum's and when we walked in we tried not to react, but we were both taken aback by how ill she looked. After spending some time with us Annie had to go to do the many jobs which could only be done on the weekend, and when she had left, there we were, the old team back together again as it had been for so many years in the past. I knew mum was very ill and as the night drew on I cooked her some dinner which she barely picked at, she just lay on the sofa which I had made into a bed for her and in her breathy voice we spoke, with me holding her hand until she finally fell off to sleep. I went into the bedroom at about midnight but left our doors open, as I lay in the dark I could hear her heavy breathing which would turn into a moan every now and then, that prompted me to keep getting up to check on her. I lay awake listening to mum till about two am when I heard her mumble something in a tortured kind of way, I leapt up and rushed into the dark living room, mum was trying to sit up and I could hardly hear what she was trying to say, she looked terrible and all I could make out were the words, want a wee wee. I helped her off of the sofa and supported her into the bathroom, she could hardly stand, I left her holding onto the sink for a moment as I lifted the toilet lid, I heard her give one deep moan and out of the corner of my eye I saw her go. She collapsed and her head went straight for the edge of the bathroom sink, thank God for martial arts honed reflexes, I will never know how but I managed to thrust my hand to her face as she hit the sink so it took the impact while my other arm was already scooping her up preventing her from hitting the floor. I was mortified but I went into automatic and lifted her into my arms and carried her like a little lifeless rag doll back into the living room and onto the sofa. As I lay her down she began to come round and I saw that she had lost all control and had wet herself upon her collapse and had continued to do so as I carried her in. She was having a fight now just to breathe so I knew I had to call an ambulance NOW.

I quickly dialled 999 and as calmly as I could gave the details and address, as soon as I got off the phone I turned back to mum who had come round enough to talk and in a weak voice she said to me, "no boy, if I go away to hospital I'll never come home", I held her hand and stroked her head saying "mum it's time for me to look after you now and I am not going to let anything happen to you, we need to get you well" she seemed to give in to me and said "o-k son", then she realised she had wet herself and that really upset her, all she could keep saying was "I'm sorry son", I changed her out of her wet clothes and as I did to help her embarrassment I said "mum how many times have you done this for me" and I gave her as brave a smile as I could. The ambulance came quickly and by the look on the crews faces when they saw her I knew mum was in a bad way. They rushed her out into the night and told me that they needed to stabilise her in the ambulance before they could attempt to take her to hospital. Right away they put her on oxygen and a heart monitor and stuck a massive needle with a drip attached into her arm, she never complained and as always put on the brave front she had always shown to the world, she looked over at my worried face and put her thumb up. After strapping her down we raced off into the night with blue lights flashing.

When we arrived at the hospital mum was rushed away from me and into intensive care, I took this chance to call Annie because no one knew all of this was going on and boy did I feel alone. I could not understand it, the line was engaged! But it was now three thirty in the morning, I tried again and again for the next couple of hours with the same result!!! I was at long last allowed into intensive care and saw my mum was now sitting up in a bed and looked a lot better, I inwardly breathed a sigh of relief, I could tell she was happy to be in safe hands being looked after and not home alone feeling unwell as she had been for some time. A nurse asked me a lot of questions about my mum including did she smoke, I said she used to but thank God she gave up fifteen years ago on my urging, they also said she was painfully thin and did I know how she got this way? I said that mum always piled on layers of clothes so we never got to see just how thin she looked underneath and I added the story about the dumps disease at which the nurse gave a strange look, then I realised she may have been hiding her weight loss for a long time because I had forgotten just when I had seen her without loads of big jumpers on. Mum was still very unwell but the spirit had returned to her eyes and she made the nurses laugh when they went to inject her by saying, "you'll never get a needle in these skinny little bastards" and held out both of her arms. People of mum's era from South

London often used swear words without ever meaning any harm, it was just a way to bolster her moral and hide her embarrassment at being so thin.

To Be Or Not To Be

I was told that mum was to be admitted and that she needed to rest and undergo some tests, so I ordered a taxi back to mums house in Long Melford, as I wound through the green lined lanes of Suffolk dawn was breaking and I was just so thankful that the long night was over and that I had been there, because mum would have died that night...alone. I had to be positive for her and the rest of my family so I had to kick myself into gear.

Back at mums house I phoned Annie again... engaged! I was starting to worry about my wife too now so I called one of my students who did not live far from us and asked him to go round and tell Annie I had spent the night trying to call her, so far I had not been able to let anyone know what had happened during that horrible night and I had rarely ever felt so alone. After some time mums phone rang and thank God it was Annie, when I told her all that had happened and how I had tried to call her she was really upset, my student (Geoff) had just called at our house telling her about the non working phone and when Annie looked she saw that the last time she used it she had not put it back on the receiver properly thus leaving the line engaged. Of all the times for this to happen, but that no longer mattered, all that was important was that Annie was ok and that she was now on her way and I would no longer have to face this alone. I also finally managed to get in contact with my sister and my two nieces Victoria and Catalina; it would need all of us together for what was to come.

Anne and I shot home to Kent so we could get ourselves together then came right back to see Mum the next day. This was a pattern we followed over the next few weeks with all of us visiting mum every chance we got including Sue and the girls. Mum seemed to be getting a bit better but she was still terribly weak and thin, with that said she was still very large in spirit, a nurse told us that on her first night in the ward she woke everyone up shouting and fighting in her sleep and even when they woke her in a confused state she still continued to shout, "Fuck off you bastard" and tried to stand up and fight them, (all six stone of her). She was so embarrassed when the nurses told her what had happened in the night, my poor old mum would not stop apologising every chance she got, all she could remember was that she had thought Martians had come to take her away and she had tried to fight them off. The lovely nurses said it was no surprise considering how ill she had been when she was admitted. All the nurses grew to love Maggie Carrigan even the male nurses, she made us all laugh and cringe at the same time when one Chinese male nurse came in and mum looked up waving her little fists in the air and shouting, Wu Hoo, Bruce Lee. My lovely little mum wasn't getting a lot better and I was really worried with a gnawing dread that she could have something terrible, not just a chest infection.

It was lunch time and I was sitting in the hospital canteen with Annie, my niece Catalina and her boyfriend who was also visiting mum, we were talking about mum's condition when I said thank God she had given up smoking all those years ago, if she hadn't I would be even more worried that she might have cancer. With that Catalina looked at me and said will you promise not to tell Nan I have told you this, I went cold and said told me what?...she forced out the words, "Nan has been smoking again for years but begged us not to tell you, it was the only way she could cope with all the stress". I slammed the table, "fuck she's killed herself". It flooded back to me, all the years I had tried to stop her because of the fear I had about her and smoking, all my arguments and pleading with her about it in Oswin Street had not been enough, I felt fear grip my insides in a way I had never known, did she have cancer? When I went back into the ward and hid how I felt from mum, I knew what she had been through and why she had turned back to those bastard things, it would hurt her so much if she knew that I had found out she had been lying to me for so long. Without her knowing I left Annie and Cat with mum and I went to find a nurse, I came right out with it, could my mother have cancer. The nurse was between a rock and a hard place, she said I can't really tell you anything...we did find something not quite right in her blood but that's all I can say, I could not end on that note, who can I talk to about this, the nurse gave me a number to call and we left it at that.

As soon as Anne and I got home I called the number and finally spoke to a doctor, again I asked the dreaded question. The doctor said I am not really supposed to talk about your mothers condition until all the results are in, but to be honest I have seen her x-rays and we would have seen something by now if she had cancer, so I think you can relax on that score but there is a possible chance that she has COPD (chronic obstructive pulmonary disease) which is the lesser of two evils. When I put the phone down I felt so relieved, COPD was bad enough but people could live for years with it as long as they were looked after, and boy would she be looked after, I would make sure that I brought her back to her beloved Kent, she deserved to be happy and safe in the place she had always loved so much. I told Sue the news and she breathed a sigh of relief with me. Mum was released and went back to her little home and Annie and I decided that we wanted to bring her down to us for a holiday and a rest. Alas it was not to be, because a few days later she had trouble breathing again and nearly collapsed so mum was taken back into hospital for more tests.

A couple of weeks went by and Annie and I were getting ready to go down and see mum when the phone rang, I picked it up and it was Sue, her voice struck me like a knife and the world spun, MUM HAS CANCER, SHE HAS THREE WEEKS TO LIVE, on hearing those words I found it hard to see, to hear and to breath. Sue said a doctor had spoken to her and said that apart from problems with her lungs mum had a massive growth on her breast bone which at first had not shown up on the x-rays, they now wanted to rush her to Addenbrooks hospital to give her chemo and radiotherapy to prolong her life and make her death easier, I said what do they mean death easier? Sue was in tears by now and said the tumour is near her heart and it could literally explode giving her a terrible death, they want to try and shrink it to help her breathe, give her maybe a few more months and ease her end. We had to decide if it was worth putting her through all of that if she was still going to die. It only took a moment; we decided anything would be worth it if it meant that she did not suffer as much when the end came. After I put the phone down I was numb, I called out to Annie and rushed up the stairs to her, as I told her the terrible news it began to hit me, I felt as if my world had come to an end, I was going to lose the person who had been everything to me my whole life, I exploded into a mass of tears and anger. Over the next few weeks especially when I was alone the feeling of total despair and helplessness would overcome me and I would turn into this werewolf crying and baying at the moon, with a mixture of rage and utter heartbreak. No one likes to lose their mothers but I suppose because of all we had been through together during the darkest days with Harry, she had come to mean so much more than just my mum.

In her heart she knew what she had but she continued to say to us, "I told the doctors I don't want to know what I have, whatever it is it can fuck off". We were not going to tell her that without treatment she had been given only weeks to live, we did tell her she needed emergency treatment to get rid of what she had so she would be able to breathe better. Mum had needed oxygen more and more as her breathing got worse and her tumour grew, sometimes she seemed to almost panic without it. We were not lying to her about her treatment helping her to breathe the only thing we kept from her was that it would only help her for so short a time.

Buying Time

In the hospital mum still tried to keep her spirits up and at one point on one of her better days she even had a woman who was in the bed next to her join in a little sing along of old London songs, but the rest of us knew that when mum went to Addenbrooks for the vital treatment. It could kill her just as surely as her illness, but to ease her suffering and give us even a few more weeks with her had to be worth the risk. We had arranged it so that all of us could be there to see her off on the day she was due to go to Addenbrooks, joining Annie and me at mums bedside were Sue, Victoria and Catalina. We also made sure that little Nathan, who mum had looked after for so long and loved so much, would also be with us to see his new nanny for what might be the last time. Mum had been too weak to walk for some time now but when she saw Nathan walk into the ward and come toward her, she got up out of the chair beside her bed on her own and held out her little fragile arms to cuddle him. It was a day I will never forget as we as we all stood around my mum with tears in our eyes and pain in our hearts. Mum reached out and we all took her hands then she said "I love all my kids", at which point she broke down too. We stayed with her and even walked beside her trolley as she was wheeled to the ambulance, goodbyes were said and the girls and Nathan walked away in tears. I stayed with my mum putting on a brave face for her, we had a kiss and a cuddle and just before the ambulance doors were closed I looked into her big blue eyes and a moment passed between us which needed no words, then as if to help me through she shot up her thumb and I did the same as I said our special battle cry, (Top of the world ma). The doors closed and she was gone, I did not know if I would ever look into those eyes again. Then it was time for a tear to trickle down my face, I did not have to be brave anymore.

We had heard that chemo and radiotherapy was very gruelling and visitors were not allowed during the sessions, but as it turned out we were wrong, a nurse told us that it is better for patients to have visitors during these times, we welcome it. That was all we needed, Annie and I were at Addenbrooks every chance we got and far from being a frightening place the floor mum was on was great. The only thing she did not like was how high up she was. Mum had a room which she shared with just two other people so that was great for us to visit her in and she had plenty of space for all the flowers she had received. By the time we got to see her mum had already been given the radiotherapy on her chest and she made sure we took a look at the cross which had been drawn on her chest to act as a target for the radiation. Mum did seem to be a lot brighter in the new hospital and looked much better in herself, but she did tell me how afraid she had been when they put her in the radiotherapy machine and she was all alone with her fears and her thoughts, but as always she toughed it out and said well whatever I've got it can piss up the wall and play with the steam, it's not going to beat me. To help keep her spirits up when we were not around I left her with a Kung Fu teddy bear which did all kinds of Kung Fu type noises when you pressed its tummy, she loved it. During one of our visits a doctor called Anne and I into a private room, he told us that the radiotherapy had been a success and they had decided not to give mum any chemo. Her chest tumour had shrunk a great deal (I dared to hope) he then said this is not a cure, we have bought your mother maybe three months at most, and she should pass away more peacefully when the end comes. Hearing those words to my face again cut like a knife, but I had vowed to myself for mum and everyone around me that I would shed no more tears till the time came. The doctor then said that mum was going back to Bury St Edmonds where she had come from and the rest was up to us.

When mum was brought back to Bury hospital she again started to become agitated and worry, she still had to have oxygen every now and again and she knew she would have a problem living on her own again because she could not walk, cook or even wash herself without help, my poor lovely old mum did not know she only had months to live. I had looked into getting her into a sheltered home in Kent not far from us (we knew that is where her heart had always been) but that had happened when we thought she only had COPD and years to live, now she only had a couple of months at best. There was only one answer, mum had to come down to Tonbridge and live with Annie and me but we could not allow her to know just how short a time that would be for. We had many things to sort out so that she could come down to us, her home had to be emptied and her furniture and belongings brought down and stored in our garage, and most importantly I had an oxygen supply to try and organise for her. It was also obvious that mum would need a lot of medical support when she came to live with us so I had to try and get my mum registered with my doctor, who luckily for me was one of the nicest people you could ever wish to meet. Little did I know that my visit to the doctor would start off a chain of events which I am still sometimes emotionally effected by even today, events not directly concerning what was happening to my lovely mum but frighteningly connected all the same.

I had been having a dry throat for months which would mainly hit me when I went to bed, my throat would begin to dry and burn, which would in turn cause my eyes to stream and then I would begin to cough. Sometimes this would also happen during the day and my voice would turn kind of gravely. The thing which really began to worry me was when I had taken a drink of water to help my coughing it had caused my throat to burn, this had happened on a couple of occasions and it had now started to nag at the back of my mind. For years I had felt my voice strain with all of my teaching and tensing of my throat during training, and I would often come home after a hard day in the club and down loads of milk to ease my throat. Now added to that was all my drama training and script reading out loud, and I had begun to notice my throat getting worse. My doctor's name was Dr Love, and she certainly lived up to her name. She was so sympathetic and understanding about my mum's situation and did not hesitate to sign her up as one of her special patients. Before I left the surgery I mentioned to her about my throat and asked her to take a look which she did, and when I told her that sometimes water made it burn she said I had better go to hospital to get it looked at. Because of mums condition the word cancer was large in my mind and I said to her it couldn't be that could it? She said that she did not think so but she could not rule out anything, which is what she was sending me to hospital for, just to be on the safe side. As I left the surgery I had a sick feeling in the pit of my stomach, I had thought about nothing but mums cancer for weeks now, and it seemed unreal that I was now going for tests to see if I had it too, my mind raced.

I still had to focus on my mum she had to be looked after and Annie and I had a lot to do to get our home ready in a very short time, but because we had to, we managed to complete our preparations for mums arrival. No sooner had we finished when I got a call to go to the hospital for my first check up. I would have done it alone but after all the stress I had been going through over mum I was very grateful when my (then) best friend for many years (Mike) offered to come with me to give his support. I was first given the dreaded blood test which was surprisingly painless and then I went in to see a doctor. She asked me some questions then sat me down in a chair and after giving me a quick once over pulled out what could only be described as a long thin silver jointed snake which turned out to be an endoscopic camera, and before I could really say anything she stuck it up my nostril and began to push. It burnt like hell as the snake like camera passed through my nose and down into my voice box. The doctor said now make a humming noise or you will want to vomit (she was so right) after looking for a while with me making my stupid humming sound, the doctor then said I have some good news and some bad news, the good news is that your voice box looks clear, the bad news is that the camera feels worse coming out than it did going in, (she was right again). My eyes and nose felt as if they were on fire. With the ordeal over she asked me if I had noticed any swelling or lumps around my neck or throat, I almost wanted to say no, but I told her that for a few months now I had felt some discomfort from a hard kind of lump near my collar bone, I showed her where and I saw her face change. Yes you do have quite a large swelling where your lymph gland should be, it could be nothing, she paused or it could be something nasty. I again felt the room spin. She then said that she would have to schedule me in for further tests but I was not to worry (fat chance). My lovely mum was coming home to die of cancer and now I had the sword of Damocles hanging over my head, the horrible word lymphoma blazed brightly across my mind. But not now, not today, I had to focus on looking after my mum and caring for her would take all I had, the rest, as mum always said, was in God's hands.

Tie A Yellow Ribbon

Mum was due to be brought all the way from Essex to Kent by ambulance which would be her last long journey. I had her oxygen ready and her bedroom waiting for her and even though my mum was technically coming home to die we would never ever let her know or feel that, after all she had been through I wanted her to have as happy a homecoming back to her beloved Kent as possible.

Years ago when we had taken over the house in Plaxtol, the song "Tie a Yellow Ribbon" had just come out, and we would play it over and over again, it had come to symbolise our homecoming back to Plaxtol and our lovely house in Kent. So I went out and bought a load of yellow ribbon along with a big yellow bow and when the day of mum's arrival came I tied it all around a lovely apple tree which we had in our front garden. As I waited for the ambulance to draw up I was filled with a mixture of fear sadness and also relief, my long suffering mum would finally be back in the place she loved and I knew that she would be looked after. As I sat on my front doorstep looking down the hill, my mind full of memories I suddenly saw the ambulance enter our road, I ran in and turned on the record player and Tony Orlando and Dawn began to sing our song. As the two ambulance men opened the back door and wheeled my frail tired mum out her eyes rested on our apple tree covered in yellow ribbon and when they carried her up the steps and into our front room she recognised the music right away and said it's our song. I kissed her and said welcome home mum, and tears rolled down her face soon to be joined by mine. Whatever lay ahead we knew that as always, we would face it together.

I'm Getting There

In my mind I thought (hoped) mum would start to get better and we would be able to have some lovely times during what time she had left and mum certainly thought she would get well and eventually be able to move into a little sheltered accommodation somewhere near us, that is why all of her furniture and belongings were now loaded into our garage. But alas those lovely times would never come.

mum had developed a fear about breathing since spending God knows how long on her own fighting for breath without telling anyone, and she would only sit for a short time now without wanting her oxygen, at first this caused a problem because I had a fear that she might run out and not have any when she really needed it. I used to try and dissuade her from using her oxygen so often till I realised how cruel it was of me to try and ration her on something so vital, when I would have given her the world if I could. I decided something had to be done so I made it my mission to order plenty of large spare cylinders, as well as small portable ones so we could travel on days out.

I knew that when mum first arrived she would be weak so we bought her a wheelchair and rigged up the portable cylinders to fit on it, and as soon as mum knew we had plenty of oxygen on hand it seemed to calm her craving for it and she went on it less during the day. I really had no idea what looking after my lovely mum would entail and in the end to be honest it almost broke me doing it. On mum's first night with us she could hardly stand but she looked up at me and smiled saying I'm getting there, I held out my arms and she did the same, I felt her frail little hands in mine as she struggled to stand, looking right into my eyes the whole time, when she finally managed to stand I scooped her up into my arms and sang the Superman theme, then as I would do many more times during her stay I carried her up the stairs to her bedroom.

Unfortunately it seemed to be the hottest summer ever and that made breathing all the harder for her, but we bought a large fan for her room and we turned it on long before she went to bed. We rigged the oxygen up beside her along with her commode and prayed she would have a good first night and sleep. As I lay in my bed I listened for her every move, I feared her getting out of bed and falling over. At about three in the morning I heard a noise coming from mum's room, I jumped up and hurried in, I saw a sight which will stay with me forever. There was my little mum squatting over a plastic oval waste paper bin peeing, we had put a plastic bin liner in the bin and I could hear it filling up as mum continued to go. I knew what a feat it must have been for her to get to the bin, she was so weak. As she squatted her big blue eyes looked at me standing in the doorway and I remember saying, "babe what are you doing..." In a shaky delirious voice she replied "sorry nurse, I pushed the button but nobody came, sorry, sorry".

She did not know where she was, the days travel and all the upheaval had made her delirious, but bless her she had not spilled a drop of pee anywhere. I helped her back to bed and cleared the bin up then I sat with her till the dawn came, It broke my heart. When mum realised what she had done in the night, she was so worried about our floor or what she had done to our bin, God bless her, but I did manage to make her laugh about it by cracking a few not so tasteful jokes about the nights events.

For a short while though mum did seem to be getting better as well as stronger, and I started to look forward to spending some happy quality time with her during the short time we had left. On one occasion I helped mum to stand so I could carry her up stairs and when she rose and stood with me still holding her hands she began to do a little dance with me and gave me a lovely smile saying I'm getting there boy. It was a lovely bittersweet moment that I will remember forever, and she even insisted that with me still holding her hands she would walk back down the stairs. I know that every slow step took all she had but showing the heart which had seen her through so many impossible moments in her life, she did it.

Her improvement meant that I got the chance to take her down into the town in her wheelchair which again filled us both with mixed emotions. Because of the sun mum wore a peak cap which Victoria had given her and with her oxygen strapped to the chair we set off. First we went food shopping in the supermarket and as we walked round who should come up to us but Karen, the girl I went with and lived with all those years ago. She hugged us and I saw how shocked she was to see my mum looking that way and as we parted I saw the tears well up in her eyes. After our food shop I took mum into a restaurant which I knew had wheelchair access. I knew that mum felt embarrassed at being wheeled about after a life spent looking after others, but as I told her, if it came to it I would gladly do it forever because the only reason I had come so far in my life was because of the sacrifice and love she had shown all through our darkest times, without her there would be no me.

The last day I had out with my mother came when Annie's mum (Pam) came to visit, we all decided to go for a trip (wheelchair and all) to the then fairly new Blue Water shopping centre, when we arrived mum said she had never seen a place like it. It was all so new to her now to see the big world outside, she had been out for shopping trips with my sister but her life for the past few years had been one of increasing isolation while she focussed on looking after little Nathan. I felt so sad and partly responsible that I had taken so long to do this, she would never get the chance again. Unfortunately mum's decline began all too soon; the 101 degree heat began to torture her as it became harder for her to breathe. Around five most mornings mum would wake and sometimes go through what are known as night terrors and panic attacks so I would get up and go in and sit with her calming her down, that is how most days would begin. The rest of the day was spent carrying mum up and down the stairs, cooking her food and trying to get her to eat, making sure she had all her medicine and tablets, constantly giving her oxygen, putting her on and off of the commode and generally trying to keep her spirits up and give her all I could. It was only when I stopped to think and sat and looked at mum that it fully sunk in, soon she would be gone and there was nothing I could do to change that, I would go away and crumble for a moment then get back to the job at hand.

During mum's time with us we had many visitors who wanted to spend as much time with her as they could, my nieces Victoria and Catalina came to spend time with us and brought little Nathan to see his new nanny, (his nickname for her). He sat for hours with his little arm around her as if he knew that this would be the last time, we also had visits from people who had known mum during her days in Plaxtol and even my ex Lynne, who I had not seen since I had walked out on her for Carol contacted us and came with her mum to see us. I thought that was a lovely brave thing to do especially after how I had treated her and broke her heart; it finally gave us the chance to lay some ghosts of our own. Mums only surviving sister Joan and her daughter Michelle also made sure they came to be with us as much as they could.

But another tragedy was that at the time she was visiting mum no one knew Michelle had a brain tumour that would also take her life months later.

At the end of the first couple of weeks of mum's stay the pressure began to show on all of us, my wife Anne was at work all day and with me only being able to teach the odd lesson because I could not leave mum on her own, it was up to Annie to keep us afloat money wise, and it was only when Victoria, Catalina or Annie's mum came down to stay for a few days that life became a little easier. I felt the weight of the world on my shoulders and sometimes I would remember that I would be going for cancer tests myself soon, which filled me with dread, then I would feel guilty about worrying about myself when my lovely mum had only a short time to live, it drove me mad. As mum began to grow weaker she had to lie down most of the time which meant she was on the sofa in the front room till bedtime when I would carry her upstairs, this all began to take its toll on Annie as well as on me.

Annie sometimes handles pressure by holding her feelings inside and puts on a seemingly tough front to the world, and her way of helping me through was to be strong all the time, which sometimes came across as uncaring, which was far from the truth. One morning when all of our pressures were at their highest and I had been up most of the night with mum we exploded. Annie was getting ready to go and see her mum and I was rushing around looking after mine. Now Annie and I love to look after and feed all the lovely garden birds and animals who had made our garden their home, and this morning Annie said to me as I rushed by, "have you fed the birds yet", and I said, "no I haven't I have got more important things to do at the moment". Whether it was the tone I used or not I don't know but Annie snapped, pushing past me and saying, "fine I'll do it like I have to do everything else around here", then she stormed into the garden and began feeding the birds. I followed and we began to argue around the garden as she filled the bird baskets, this continued as she came back in and headed for the door to leave for work and we reached fever pitch. I snapped, "my mum is dying upstairs and all you can think about is my feeding the birds, FUCK THE BIRDS" Annie stepped forward shouting back at me then she pushed me in the chest,...I reacted and shoved her back by pushing her shoulders against the door. We had a moment of stunned silence then she stormed out in tears and I just stood there shaking before my own tears started to stream down my face. I was going to lose my mother and now (in a different way) maybe my wife too. These really were the worst of times. Annie had been fantastic in so many ways and she was under tremendous pressure holding the home together and paying the bills while I became a carer, but she could never know how I really felt inside watching someone I loved so much crumble bit by bit, day by day, having no sleep, constantly tending mum, and also deep inside thinking, this could all be in store for me if it turns out that I have cancer too…almost unbearable.

The Final Journey

When Annie came home we had to talk, so we got all of our feelings out in the open. It turned out that Annie had a terrible fear of my mum dying in our home; she said that if she did she would not be able to live there any longer. She also said that mum was now so ill that she was beyond my looking after but I could not see it. In my heart I knew that she was right, the nurses who visited mum to wash her were fantastic, but they could only visit a few times a week, and now mum really had become a full time job. I had to lift her everywhere now and the last straw had really been when she did not have the strength to wipe herself after she had been to the toilet, which is something no mother and son should ever have to be put through, she was terribly ill but she still had her dignity and I was not just her carer, I was still her son.

I knew the time had come, I had looked after my darling mum for a month now but I knew she was suffering and was beyond just my help. It was so hard to do but I sat on the sofa and said to mum that the nurses had told me she could go to the hospice for respite, to help her get strong again and also to give me a rest. I saw her face when she heard the word hospice and it broke my heart, she knew what a hospice really meant and maybe in her heart she knew what she had, but we never said the word cancer or talked about dying. The only time we had shared any kind of despair was while we were watching TV one day alone together and Harry Neilson came on singing his hit song called 'Without You', we sat in silence holding hands, and at one point we turned to each other and tears began to role down our cheeks, we automatically just reached out and held onto each other and began to sob. We both knew why but never said. After I had spoken to her about the hospice she just looked into my eyes and almost resignedly said, "Ok boy, I'll do it for you".

After talking to mum it was with a heavy heart and a lump in my throat that I phoned my doctor, as I have said before she was a lovely person and arranged to come round right away. When she arrived the first thing she did was to give mum a hug and then proceeded to do her best to put all mums fears to rest. They even started to talk about all the old hop picking days which mum had loved so much, but mum would keep going back to saying, "if I go into a hospice I will never come out again will I?". Doctor Love took me to one side and saw how hurt I was at not being able to keep mum with me; I felt I had let her down. The doctor held my hand and said, "You have done a fantastic job, now we have to do ours". Because there was such a waiting list for the twelve or so hospice beds mum would have to be assessed by the head doctor from the hospice first. We only had a few hours to wait before an elderly lady arrived, you could tell by her strength of character that she was someone who had seen it all before and knew her job well. She sat on the sofa beside mum and said right away, "you are poorly aren't you? We want you to come and have a rest with us so we can put some meat back on you, help you breathe and get strong enough to come home again, is that ok with you?. Your son and daughter in law have done a wonderful job but we have the specialist care you need right now". My lovely old mum God bless her shrugged her shoulders and just said, "Whatever you want to do". I knew then that inside she had given up hope. The doctor took me to one side and said to me, "your mother is painfully thin and she is just the kind of case who needs our help, we will take over now". A wave of mixed feelings flooded over me, I felt a great sense of relief that we were no longer on our own looking after mum, but I also felt as if I had let her down and was almost abandoning her, which is something she had never done to my sister and I during all our troubled nearly impossible times. We arranged for Annie and I to take her to the hospice that very day, it was to be her final journey.

I sat with my mum in the back of the car holding her hand and as we drove I told her that this was just to make her strong again, it broke my heart when she looked at me and said, "you will visit me won't you?" This was my mum, the centre of my world and I would have gone to the end of the universe to see her if I had to. As I said, taking her to the hospice broke my heart but I knew it was a blessing too. When we arrived I was so relieved to see that The Hospice in the Weald (as it was called) was a lovely modern place surrounded by countryside, and all the patients had lovely large rooms of their own with a patio which led to a lovely garden. I noticed right away just how caring all the doctors and nurses were, not only with the patients but also with the families who were there to visit them, in fact during one of my first few visits I was taken into a room by a really nice male nurse who spoke to me to see if I needed counselling over what we had been through and what we were about to go through. During our conversation he picked up on the fact that after all of my years of inward searching through the martial arts I did seem to have a strong inner core and was holding up ok.

Mum began to settle down and in fact grew to love the hospice and the nurses, she grew particularly close to a nurse called Lindy, Lindy said to me what a lovely lady your mum is and then added, what a character, she was right on both counts. The hospice was almost luxury compared to what mum had been used to most of her life, she was really looked after. The gardens overlooked hop fields and strawberry fields and one day I took mum around the gardens in her wheelchair, we saw people in the distance picking strawberries and suddenly mum turned to me and said, "Take me inside love". I saw that she was crying, I bent down to her and asked what was wrong. She said that the people picking in the fields reminded her too much of the life she once had in Plaxtol, a life, her life which was now over. I knew just what the hopping and fruit picking days had meant to her so later that day I went down the road and onto a farm where I had seen a hop sign, I found the farmer and explained about my mum. Then I asked if I could buy a large sprig of hops from him, he said, "No son but you can take them as a gift from me". I was really moved by the look on his face as I gathered up an armful of hops and set off at a run back to the hospice. I walked into mum's room and placed the hops in her arms, she held them to her face and her eyes filled up as she said, "its me hopping smell".

Mum had a lot of visitors again while she was in the hospice, including more old friends from Plaxtol, Victoria, Catalina and Aunt Joan with Michelle, and I was really pleased when my ex Lynne started to make regular visits to see her, as she said to mum one day, "I was nearly your daughter in law Maggie and you were like my second mum". I was not sure how Annie would react to Lynne but thank God she loved her, and at one point in the gardens away from mum they hugged and cried in each others arms.

The only person I really wished had seen more of mum during those last days was her daughter, my sister Sue. Sue had lived around the corner from mum in Suffolk and they were together a lot for years, but over the months leading up to mum's illness they had grown apart. Part of the reason for their distance was Sue's boyfriend, who for want of a better word was a right bastard. We had learned that he had hit her a couple of times and mum like me, hated him. I just wanted to knock him out for what he had done to my sister but it seemed that Sue wanted him, so what could anyone do. So it was that Sue only got to see mum once during her time in the hospice and he came with her, we all just gritted our teeth (including my mum) and I used to wonder what Harry boy would have done to him if he had been here. I know Sue now regrets not seeing mum during those sad days, but we can't change the past, we all have things we would have done differently given the gift of hindsight.

As the first week drew to a close we began to see a change in mum, a change for the worst, a doctor took me aside and said, "your mother knows in her heart what illness she has, but she has such a spirit she will not give in or admit what is going to happen, she just says to us I don't want to know. In some ways that can be a good thing but it can also leave so much unsaid, then it is too late, I think it is time you had the mother and son talk, say all you want to say". With a lump in my throat like I had never known and fighting back the tears I went into mum's room alone. I sat on her bed and took her hand, then I said, "me old mum I need to tell you something, I love you more than anything in this world but this is one fight you can't win, this illness will take you from me and there is so much I need to say to you". Mum looked at me with her blue eyes and said, "I know son, I know". Then the tears overwhelmed us and we just held on to each other like there was no tomorrow, because for us there wasn't. We had the long mother and son talk which would have to last us for eternity, it was our last time alone together, just the two of us as it had always been.

She's Gone

The last lovely night we shared with mum saw Annie and I around mums bed with Victoria and Catalina beside us, mum was tired but in good spirits and I knew she was doing it for us, as always.

Victoria and Catalina were red faced and puffy eyed from too many tears, we had all hugged kissed and cried on and off all day with mum making us smile between the tears with her cockney spirit but she kept on drifting off into fits of sleep. At one point she had her eyes shut but was pointing her fingers up and down in the air, I had seen her do it many times during her life, it was part of a dance from the 1940s called The Truck, her eyes opened and she gave us a lovely smile, then she turned to me and said, "I was trucking with Harry". As night drew on and we were all around her bed a moment came which gave all of us a lasting memory of the woman she was. My mum turned to me and looked me right in the eyes, then pointed to me saying, "live love laugh and be happy", she then pointed at Annie and said, "live love laugh and be happy". She went around the bed giving each one of us that lovely look in the eyes followed by those words; we all had eyes full of silent tears. The doctors had told us that she was very weak now and could pass away that night so we all elected to stay at the hospice. While the rest tried to get some sleep in any spare rooms or in the lounge I stayed beside mum's bed in a chair, it was one of the longest nights you could imagine but as dawn came mum was still with us. It was hard for them but the girls had to go back to Suffolk for work and when the time came they left in floods of tears.

Up to this point thankfully mum had been in little or no pain and her oxygen had helped her to breathe, but this time when she woke she began to suffer pain in her stomach so she had to be given an automatic morphine dispenser which gave her a regular controlled infusion, thank God this did seem to help. I was so glad when mums sister, my Aunt Joan turned up to be with us, but it was not a good day. Mum's pain began to increase which drove me mad I did not want her to suffer. Mum continued to drift in and out of her deep coma like sleep. As we held her hands, but at one point she woke up and began to call out in pain, I knew how bad the pain must have been because she called out. "Nurse help me it hurts, God help me don't let me wake up". I ran for the nurse who came and she was already on the maximum morphine dose they could give her. Mum reached out to me and said "cuddle", I bent down and held her and she whispered to me, "I love you son", I whispered back "I love you mum, all the world and even more". I lay her back and stroked her hair till she fell thankfully back into her deep sleep; she stayed that way for the rest of the day. By tea time my Aunt Joan had left and a nurse said to Annie and I that we should nip home for a change of clothes and a meal, she would make sure that we were informed right away if mums condition changed. We had been in the hospice for days now so we agreed and said we would be back in a couple of hours. When we got home we rushed to bath and change and were just about to grab a snack when the phone rang, it was the hospice, you had better get back as fast as you can (the same words I had heard about my father a few years before). We flew into the car and back to the hospice, when we got to mums room I was so pleased to see that my lovely ex, Lynne had turned up out of the blue and had been sitting with my mum. We all knew the end was close so Lynne hugged us and said I will leave you two alone with Maggie now, then she left.

Annie and I sat down and prepared for the night to come, the evening continued with Annie dozing in a chair and me sitting holding mums hand and whispering to her how much I loved her and telling her she was going to a lovely place to be with her Harry. Each time she drew a deep breath I held mine until she breathed out again. After a couple of hours I saw what I thought was a large moth whiz past my eyes, but when I turned to follow it there was no sign, I also seemed to see some kind of white mist hanging in one corner of the room, was it my imagination or something more? I had sat beside mum holding her hand for hours now and my legs told me I needed to move, I whispered to mum that I would not be a moment and I got up and walked across the room. After a moment I turned around to look over at mum and it hit me, her eyes had opened, I rushed over to her and bent down close looking right into her eyes and I said, "Hello babe". With that her mouth opened and one long breath came out, then all was still...I froze for a moment and then called to Annie, "she's gone". We stayed in silence looking at her for a long time (or so it seemed) then I went to tell a nurse that it was over. When we finally forced ourselves to leave I held myself together till we got into the car, then the floodgates opened and the dam burst.

The days that followed were filled with confusion tears and all the red tape you have to go through following a death while you have to (as they say) put their affairs in order. It turned out that my darling mum old mum had just one pound and fifty pence in her building society when she died and no money anywhere to pay for her funeral. I did remember her paying into a funeral scheme for many years but what had become of it I had no idea. Annie and I decided to re-mortgage to pay for her funeral and consolidate all our debts. It was not until nearly two weeks later that my mum was ready to be viewed at the funeral parlour, which was really too long. I felt I owed it to mum to see her so I went on my own, I wish now that I had not, because I find it hard to shake that last vision of her from my mind. It was not the woman I knew and was not at all like the lovely last look I had of my father, but I had to be with her one last time to say goodbye, just the two of us, as we had always been.

During our last mother and son talk my mum had told me that she wanted to be cremated and her ashes were to stay with Annie and me in her beloved Kent, my sister Sue had told me that some time ago mum had said to her, when I die I don't want to be buried with your father, if I hadn't married him you and John wouldn't have had the tortured life you went through. All our lives were ruined; I don't want to be with him. Sue said mum felt racked with guilt, as if it was all her fault. Mum may have said that to Sue during a down day when she was filled with remorse, but if I know anything in this life it is that mum loved her Harry more than anyone can ever know. During her trauma filled life with the man she married she had many offers and chances to leave him, but she stuck fast no matter what and when his life was falling apart around him he knew that his Maggie would always be there. Whatever mum said or felt, I know she loved him till the end of her days. Anne and I were determined to give my mum the funeral she deserved, to do justice to the woman she was. The wreath I had made for her was laced with hops because her young days as a hop picker were the happiest days of her life, and all the rest of the flowers were spring and summer colours to celebrate how she lived, not how she died. Mum is now in her own special place in our garden with her own angel statue to watch over her and on a little stone in gold writing are the words she used to say when things seemed at their darkest, "If God don't come he sends" and we make sure that she is always surrounded by lovely bright flowers. Every day when I go out to feed the birds and squirrels I say hello to the little lady I owe everything to, "Maggie Carrigan" my mum.

The Test

The day before mums funeral I received a letter which had been delayed in the post telling me that I had to go for my cancer test on the very day of the funeral, which meant I had to quickly phone up and explain the situation, they were very understanding and quickly rescheduled my appointment for a few days later. As you can imagine my insides were torn up over mum already so when the time came for my appointment I was filled with nothing but dread. I had been told that I was going to have an ultra sound followed by something called a deep needle exploratory into my neck, just the name alone made me want to head for the hills.

Once in the hospital I stripped off for the ultra sound and a doctor began to run a scanner over my neck while he stared at a monitor, after a few moments he started to say to himself, "Yes I see, mmm I see". I thought oh no he has found something, he then continued "in your notes it says that you practice martial arts, can you show me something", I thought what ?? He then said, "you know an action you do a lot with your right arm"?? So I did a lead right hand punch, he said "ah ha, do it again and hold the pose", so I did. He smiled and said "I was going to do a deep needle exploratory on you but I have no need to do it now". I breathed a sigh of relief, he then said "you have developed an extra muscle right over your lymph gland which should not really be there,

I have never come across this before, it looks as if it is all due to that punching action. I will have to make up a new name for it maybe I will call it the Incredible Hulk syndrome". He then added there is no sign of a tumour, well done. I was over the moon but I would still have to go for what was called a barium swallow.

I walked into my second test with my hopes a little higher and was told to swallow what looked like white paint, radioactive paint at that. I stood on a platform which tipped up and down as the scanner scanned my entire body, when it was over I stood and held my breath. The doctor came out from behind his shielded position and called me over saying "I have some good news and some bad news" (my heart missed a beat). "The good news is that there is no sign of anything bad in your body, (I did an inner smile) but I can see that you have had multiple fractures to your body over time, how has this happened?" I explained all about the martial arts and stunt work, he then said "well the bad news is that you have spondylitus of the spine, mainly in the third vertebra, when did you fracture your neck?" I said "what!! I didn't!" Then I realised he must be talking about my stair fall stunt which went wrong a few years ago. The doctor continued, "You were very lucky you could have completely broken your neck". As it was it was only a partial fracture, (a nearly broken neck and I never knew), he then said "you must get a great deal of back pain and I would be surprised if you can touch your toes with your back fusion". I said I did get quite a lot of back pain but I had just put that down to my over training, and as for touching my toes. I then put my palms to the floor and my head on my knees before dropping into the splits. The doctor grinned and said, "You are a very unusual person, normally the only thing we can suggest for a condition like yours is physio to try and ease the symptoms but it looks as if your life is one constant physio, so carry on doing what your doing, but no more broken bones ok?" I was given the all clear, no sign of cancer, but I had an extra muscle and spondylitus, I could live with that, what a bargain. It felt as if the clouds were finally lifting, my darling mum was gone but I was determined to live my life to the full, for myself, my mum and my dad, if only I had known what lie in store.

You Only Live Twice

Time marched on and I tried to adjust to life without mum, I also tried to live up to the promise I had made myself to live life to the full and appreciate every day, and to a certain degree I did. Although I had always been a positive person I had spent most of my life worrying about when the rain would fall, so I would never really appreciate the sun. That part of me was changing but it was still too soon and the loss of mum would ambush me sometimes when I least expected it, I even had a strange experience which may or may not have been a visit from my mum. I had been training and came home after a long day, Annie was not yet in. I had no thoughts of mum in my mind at the time and I was perched on the sofa taking off my training shoes. All of a sudden I sprang to my feet and spun around in a fighting stance, out of the corner of my eye, a person in blue right beside me, as I turned they were gone? After I had calmed down I was annoyed at myself for reacting the way I did, the one wish in all the world would have been to see mum again, and what did I do, jump up ready to fight. I will never know what or who it was but I will always wonder.

It was nearly a year now since mum had passed away and I had missed two filming parts which I had really wanted, one of which had been after a gruelling four hour audition. It was August 2004 and I had been teaching and training hard and not really living up to my new totally positive vibe way of life. It had been a hard day and I really needed a recharge and a soak in the bath. As I lay there contemplating the universe I felt a small lump at the top of my groin, I thought oh shit I have a hernia, then all the ways I could have got it flashed through my mind, but all I could think of was that a student had missed the kick pad a week before and caught the exact spot where I had the lump. I then continued feeling my testicles just to make sure, a shock hit me as I felt yet another lump on my left testicle. All the feelings of dread and fear from the year before came flooding back, not again. I went straight to the doctors the next day, I almost felt embarrassed to be going back again with yet more lumps, as if I thought they might think I was imagining all of this or something (if only).

My lovely doctor had now moved on so I had to see my new doctor for the first time, I did not fancy dropping my pants on our first meeting but it had to be. I told her I thought I had a hernia and almost did not tell her about my second lump but I relented and pointed that out too. She examined me and I tensed up dreading her words. "Well I am afraid it is not a hernia it is an enlarged lymph gland which could be nothing and could have reacted to the kick or it could be a warning that you have something wrong". I said "could it be cancer? She said it could be. She then felt my testicle and said; "well I am afraid this should not be there either". I can't explain how I felt, I had been through all of this before, all the weeks of worry and torment but I had got my life back, surely not again. She said "you need to go into hospital to have the gland removed for biopsy and the other lump scanned, especially with your mother's history, but we won't know what we are dealing with till then". I walked back from the doctors in a daze, it was the same month a year ago when my doctor had told me I needed to go to hospital for cancer tests on my throat and neck, now I was to have surgery this time to see if I had cancer, it was a nightmare, the whole of last year was a nightmare which I had survived, it could not be happening again. I waited for Annie to come home and told her the bad news, she was great and told me I would be fine, she said you are far too healthy to have cancer it will be nothing, I was not convinced. As the days passed and I waited for the letter from the hospital something began to happen to me. The anniversary of mum's death was just days away and everything I had been writing in this book began to come into my thoughts, I had written the upbeat ending to this book with my positive attitude after mums passing and all that, then all of a sudden I was convinced I had cancer just like my mum, the book was wrong, no happy ending. If God was really up there why was all of this happening again, I could not believe how my faith was disappearing, how the positive attitude I had always tried to live by and tried to pass on to my students was gone. I felt ashamed of myself but the demons of despair and negativity were smashing into me, all I could think was that losing mum to that bastard disease and at the same time thinking I had it last year had marked my resolve more than I realised, I was convinced I could not escape again.

As the days turned into weeks I put a brave face to the world (as us Carrigans had always done) but inside I was afraid, not only for me but also for my lovely Annie, I did not want her to be alone. It had been a month now and I still had heard nothing so I phoned the hospital and to my shock they had never received the letter from my doctors, it had been lost in the post. They took my details and promised me an urgent appointment. A whole month had been lost now and if I did have cancer time would be of the essence. I had made up my mind that my family had been fated, not to have the happy ending I had first wanted for my dad, then my mum, now it seemed that I might be denied it too. This feeling I had was completely opposite to how all of my family (including me) had lived, I was not about to give up but I could not find one positive thought for the future.

My appointment came through three days later and I went to have my first examination. After feeling all of my bits the doctor said he would book me in for surgery, he told me that the operation could be done under local anaesthetic but he would advise against it because they would have to go deep into my groin and in his words, I would not like to be awake during that myself. So it was decided they would put me to sleep when the time for my op came. I then went for an ultra sound scan on the lump in my testicles which was the other half of the worry in my mind, lymph cancer, testicular cancer, or both. With all the machines and tables I had been on I was beginning to feel like James Bond when he was strapped to the table and the bad guy says, you only live twice Mr Bond. Thank God I was given the result right away, the lump on my testicles turned out to be a non malignant cyst which would not cause me any problems and was unrelated to the lump in my groin, (phew). One down one to go.

A couple more weeks passed and all that mum had gone through haunted me, not knowing if I were next was driving me mad. As the time came for my surgery I called my martial arts club together and passed the reigns to my co-instructors, because whatever the outcome I knew it would be some while before I could jump around again. Even if they found nothing this would still be an operation which would take time to get over especially for someone who had to be able to kick over six feet in height whenever he wanted to, but I also wondered if I ever would again. Annie took me to the hospital at 8 in the morning and after a couple of hours I sent her home, I wanted to face this myself. All the long weeks of worry, doubt, fear and negativity were suddenly swept away as the real me seemed to step forward again, I faced what was to come as if it were one of the many martial arts fights I had faced in the past, the bravado and wit my mum had always shown kicked in. The surgeon met with me and said we have decided to do the operation with a local injection only, I don't think we need to put you right out and that way you can go home tonight instead of being kept in. I told him the views the other surgeon had about being too deep for a local but the doctor insisted and said I am sure we will be fine with a local injection. I said "ok I trust your judgment; I will be awake for the surgery".

As I was wheeled to the theatre I felt as all people do at the thought of being cut open (not good) but I was glad that the long wait was over and at last this hurdle was about to be jumped. As I got close to the theatre doors one of the nurses asked if I was ok, and I said "fine, just cut my leg off and give me a patch and a crutch I am sure there are plenty of pirate roles I could do". In the theatre I turned into my old gritty self, they asked if I was allergic to anything and I replied, "Only big needles", the surgeon then said, "Well I am afraid you are out of luck", he then produced the biggest needle I had ever seen. I was literally stuck to the table by a large sticky back plastic sheet which just had a square cut in to reveal my private parts and they also attached a pad to my leg which would earth me so they could seal the vessels with an electronic kind of laser. (At this point I wished I were unconscious) then without any kind of numbing cream or spray that big needle was plunged into my groin (wow) I think I might have said the F word, boy did that hurt.

I was grateful as a cold flood dispersed through my groin and any pain faded. I stared up at the large light above me as the surgeon asked, "can you feel this?". I said no (thank God) and he began his work. I spoke to the nurses and the doctors as they proceeded, ranging from the wonderful job they did to the martial arts and my film career (somehow they already knew). I did not want to look down but from time to time I saw smoke rise from my groin area as they sealed off blood vessels as they went. Then the surgeon stopped and said I have located the lymph node and I am going to remove it now, I thought I was imagining but I could swear I felt something, then...the world exploded into white light as I shouted "STOP"! As he had begun to cut the node I felt everything, it was fully alive. The doctor was shocked and quickly said I am so sorry I have had to go far deeper than I had at first anticipated and obviously the local injection has not penetrated far enough. The nurse had to go and prepare another injection which only took under a minute but with a half cut lymph gland inside me it felt like an eternity. My martial arts training really helped because I am used to pain, but pain from the outside in not the inside out, it was horrendous. The new injection took hold right away and the pain was replaced by freezing cold. As the operation drew to a close the doctor held up the offending lymph gland to show me (yuk) it was about the size of a large peanut. I was released from hospital a few hours later with a large amount of pain killers (thank goodness) and

Annie drove me home. When my groin came back to life I was in a lot of pain with stitches inside and out, but it was over thank God.

For the next two weeks I was very limited to how I could move and that meant mainly lying on my back, which for someone as active as me was not easy. My friends and students had been very supportive and of course my wife Annie had been my rock, but I had seen that my constant negative worrying had got her down so I tried to keep most of my doubts and fears to myself.

My mum had always said, if God don't come he sends and this time he really did. Not long before I went into hospital a new student arrived at my martial arts school for private lessons, her name was Kym. She was tall slim with long blond hair and was a life coach, she was also very spiritual with a strong belief in God, she picked up on the way I was feeling (although I tried to hide it) and made it her job to be a great support to me during these worrying times which helped take the burden off of Annie and gave me someone else to talk to about my inner struggles. I had waited two and a half weeks to hear my results and I could wait no more, I needed to know, I had to know. So I could get on with focusing my energy and kicking the ass of what ever it was I might have. After a phone call to the hospital the results were faxed to my doctor who then in turn called me. Faith is really built on something you can't always prove, and I had always had faith, but I have to admit by now my faith was unsure. I steeled myself as the doctor said; "you have the all clear, no sign of cancer, the node may have reacted to the kick you received which caused an infection, you can relax now Mr Carrigan". Unless you have been through this you will not know how I felt, but if you won the lottery that would be a tenth of the joy I felt. Through my life like many others I have seen more than my share of sadness and pain and if we survive that pain we come through stronger than before, but sometimes we stumble and fall-getting up again is what counts.

The Impossible Dream

I spent time recovering from my surgery and really re-evaluating my approach to life, I finally now had a grasp on what really matters in life, health and love have to be top on the list and I did and do really appreciate every sunrise. But being human my goals and dreams still burnt strong inside of me, I had climbed many mountains and I was grateful for that but I was beginning to almost give up now on my dream of ever getting anywhere in the film or TV industry. I had tried and tried and given up so much in pursuit of that dream and after all, I was not getting any younger, maybe I would never make it. I had just lost a part in a TV series which I really wanted to be in and it seemed to me that I had just about had my last chance of getting anywhere.

It was not long to go to my birthday so we decided to go away and celebrate it by doing something I had long wanted to do. We booked a trip to Seattle to visit the grave of Bruce Lee. Bruce and his teachings had given me so much in my life and it was something I felt I had to do, we also arranged to drop by LA for a couple of days to see some of our friends, after all we had been through during the past months we really needed to get away. Little did we know that fate and the Bruce Lee/Star Trek connection was about to join forces in a fantastic way.

It was Mothers Day so I was feeling down and sat lost in memories. Annie was on the computer checking our flights for the trip when she called down to me. I ran up the stairs to see an email which was from a friend of ours, Doug Drexler. Doug was an Oscar winning make up artist and CGI expert who worked on Star Trek in Hollywood. The email said urgent, call me right away we have been trying to reach you by phone but must have the wrong number. So I dashed back down stairs and called Doug. He was full of excitement and told me that a company was going to produce a new Star Trek series for the internet with the help of the fans, and one of the producers was the son of the legendary Star Trek creator Gene Roddenberry, who I had got to know all those years ago. The series was going to be set back in Captain Kirk's era with all the original sets and costumes recreated down to the last detail, but the best was yet to come. They were looking for cast members and would like me to meet the producer and director in LA to try out for a part. To be in a recreation of the original Star Trek would be like a dream come true for me and it really was fate because the meeting had been scheduled when we would already be in LA before our Bruce trip.

Annie and I jetted off a couple of days later and when we eventually met the group from Star Trek New Voyages (as the series was to be called) they were a fantastic bunch of people. Doug had vouched for me as an actor so after our meeting I was offered the part of commander Kargh of the Klingon Empire. They had seen what I had done in Advanced Warriors and they also liked the way my training made me carry myself, as they said (very upright like a warrior). After LA and then a very emotional trip to see Bruce Lee's final resting place I came home over the moon not really believing this was happening, the call had come on Mothers Day, I knew she was giving me the thumbs up from heaven.

The day soon came when it was time for me to boldly go where I had only dreamed of going before. This incarnation of Star Trek was only possible because of one fan (James Cawley). He had spent ten years and all his earnings as an Elvis tribute artist painstakingly recreating the original sets of the Starship Enterprise and it was James who had set in motion this fantastic chain of events. I arrived in Upstate New York where the sets were and everything about this trip was new to me. The starship sets were incredible and so were all of the people I would be working with. I met Eugene Roddenberry (Rod) for the first time and I swapped stories about the times I spent with his father, and I was proud that a bond of friendship grew between us. When it finally came time for me to film, I put on my Star Trek uniform and walked onto the bridge of the Starship Enterprise; I looked at Captain Kirk's chair then lowered myself into it. Many times I had sat for hours in my home made Captain's chair all those years ago in Oswin Street, trying to escape all the sadness which could be invoked by the other side of Harry when he was at his worst, wishing I could be on the Enterprise far away in some distant time and galaxy, now years later here I was. In a way I had done it, an impossible dream come true. But I was no longer the lost boy dreaming, I was the man, the actor and I had done it, but the boy inside me still was now grinning ear to ear. I had another moment on the set which was almost overwhelming. I was in full Starfleet uniform ready to beam down to a planet during a scene, I looked up to see Rod Roddenberry looking at me, he grinned and held up his thumb to me as if he knew how I was feeling and it again hit me what this show had meant to me in the past and how Rod's father had inspired me to follow my dreams, and now here I was, finally a part of Star Trek for real. I had to snap myself out of it otherwise I could never have acted the part with all of that going on inside me.

The impossible dream did not stop there. After filming my first episode I had an idea for a story which could involve bringing back Chekov (my friend Walter Koenig) at the age he looks today. The producers loved the idea but they did not know if Walter would like to be involved in this recreation of his Star Trek (they had recast all the other roles with new young actors). I sent Walter a copy of the episode I had filmed and he was very impressed, then I told him my idea for bringing him back to Star Trek and he loved it. So Walter and I finally got to work together, on of all things Star Trek. Walter had a great time and did a fantastic job and the first time he stepped back onto the set in his Starfleet uniform the whole production just erupted into spontaneous applause. I also got my lovely Annie involved with the episode and after giving her acting lessons for weeks before the shoot she got to be my Klingon first officer Le'ak as well as a blue skinned alien Ambassador.

During a quiet moment on the set I went off and sat inside a full size mock up of a shuttlecraft not unlike the one I made inside my old Star Trek room all those years ago, and I just sat sharing all these wonderful feelings with the memories of mum and dad. I had made it for them and I knew they were with me. My great impossible dream has gone from strength to strength. I am now a regular guest star on Star Trek New Voyages and I have also had a part on a 40th anniversary Star Trek tribute movie made by another production company called "Star Trek of Gods And Men", which included Walter and over a dozen other stars from past Star Trek Series and films. I never dreamed that my impossible dream would come true, I am not just on screen world wide but I am in Star Trek, who would have thought it. Top of the world Ma.

Faith

The life I led growing up left many demons inside me which have to be fought sometimes daily, doubts, always trying to prove myself, with fear of failure being top of the list. This is the legacy of the other side of Harry which I know has left my sister with her own set of demons. Looking inward I see myself clearly now as someone who always tries to make up for the lost boy I used to be, that's why I look after lost boys of my own both inside and outside of my club. I am not Peter Pan but I aspire to be Pan like. I will always try to help anyone who may feel alone in a hopeless situation, as I used to feel. Thank God I had my mum, some people have no one but their faith, some people do not even have that.

What do I believe in? A big test of faith was when I lost my father through Alzheimer's; I could not bring myself to pray for over a year. As a family although we were not regular church goers we all had a strong belief in God and many times during our troubled life all we had to turn to for help was God and prayer, all throughout our troubles my mum's faith had been especially unshakable. But when we lost our Harry I could not see how he could have come through all his years of schizophrenia and then when at last it seemed to leave him in peace so he could spend his twilight years with his Maggie as the man she fell in love with, he was again cursed this time by Alzheimer's.

I was as much heartbroken for mum as I was for dad, so for a while I lost faith. In time I came to accept what had happened and that maybe at last dad was in a place where he could truly be free and happy, and in that same way although she loved him dearly mum could now finally be free too without giving the rest of her life to looking after Harry, she had been a carer long enough. Then the bombshell of my life when mum fell ill with cancer and I had cancer scares of my own. First I prayed that mum would get well, then I had to face the fact that she would not, so I prayed that she would go to sleep peacefully. I prayed for myself during my first cancer scare, and I learned to see mum's passing as her way to finally know peace and be with her Harry again. I still held onto my faith, but then again I was thrown into turmoil and my belief was shaken by my second cancer scare in as many years. I prayed but inside for some reason I had all but lost faith, I lost dad, I lost mum and now I was sure it was my turn, like our whole life had been an amazing film with a terrible sad ending, no cavalry coming over the hill to save the day. But at the last moment in hospital it hit me again, that thing called faith and I said to myself God has not brought me this far to end my story like this, and I was right I am fine.

I do believe we go somewhere when we die, we do not end. I know my mum and dad are together again and at last they are happy. I do not know if the being is called God, Jehovah, or one of a hundred other names we know him by, I just believe that the good we do on earth lives on after we die, and somewhere in a lovely place so do we.

Closing

This whole book has been written firstly as a tribute to my mum and dad, who through no fault of their own had to make the best of the terrible hand they were dealt, but I have also written this as a testament that you CAN make it through the rain, but boy does it take determination and faith. It also takes letting go of the past, not using it as an excuse for tomorrow's failures but as a reason for today's victories, because if you let it, the past can destroy the present and the future.

Remember the thing which makes a star bright is the darkness which surrounds it; we have to learn that sometimes our darkness can also be our reason to shine. If I had been given a normal father and had what might be considered a more normal up bringing, I might have ended up with a nice wife and a house and maybe two point four children which would have been all well and good, but all the things we went through living with the other side of Harry shaped who I am today, for good and for bad, and directly because of those things the path of my life was laid out, not always through choice but sometimes out of necessity. I became a so called martial arts expert which led hundreds of people to turn to me over the years and put a big part of their life in my hands. I also chose what might be considered an unusual path given my background and character, and I became an actor who would eventually go to Hollywood and work alongside his childhood heroes, which is the stuff many so called ordinary peoples dreams are made of.

The curse of my father's illness forced me to turn my stumbling blocks into stepping stones and over the years I have actually had many people say to me, I wish I was you, which still makes me want to pinch myself to see if I am awake. I hope that you can gain something positive from my family's story and let it help you make it through your personal storms if they come along. While I have been researching this book there have been days when it has taken me back to some good times but it has also dragged me back to many bad ones, and I have found myself feeling just like the young boy I used to be with all the fears and insecurities that haunted me then, and reliving the passing of first my dad and then mum brought me to tears and left me in deep wells of depression. Writing this book has helped me to discover something I did not fully realise although I have spoken about it many times in my quest to help people with their demons, and that is just how deeply memories and feelings of days gone by can effect the present if we choose to live them over and over again in our hearts and minds. Living in the past is not always a good thing, we must remember to only visit those times, not dwell there and let them impact on today as is so easy to do. Walk on to the brightness of tomorrow.

John Carrigan

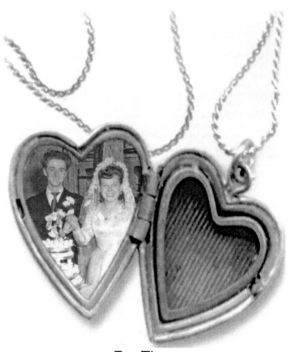

For Them